The Framingham Study

This volume is published as part of a long-standing cooperative program between Harvard University Press and the Commonwealth Fund, a philanthropic foundation, to encourage the publication of significant scholarly books in medicine and health.

The Framingham Study
The Epidemiology of Atherosclerotic Disease

Thomas Royle Dawber

A Commonwealth Fund Book

Harvard University Press
Cambridge, Massachusetts
and
London, England
1980

Library of Congress Cataloging in Publication Data

Dawber, Thomas Royle, 1913-
   The Framingham study.

   "A Commonwealth Fund book."
   Bibliography: p.
   Includes index.
   1.   Atherosclerosis—Massachusetts—Framingham.
2.   Atherosclerosis—Massachusetts—Framingham—
Statistics.   3.   Epidemiology.   I.   Title.   [DNLM:
1.   Arteriosclerosis—Occurrence.   WG550 D269f]
RC692.D38   614.5'912   80-11189
ISBN 0-674-31730-0

Preface

PHYSICIANS ARE ALMOST ENTIRELY concerned with the care of patients who present symptoms and signs of real or imaginary disease. The outcome of such disease is of utmost importance and is the subject of intensive research aimed at determining whether the course of the disease can be modified favorably. Efforts are constantly exerted to make possible earlier diagnosis, in the hope that the disease can then be modified to extend life and lessen complications and disability.

The concept of expanding our interest in the patient beyond the onset and course of the disease is not new. Over the years the desirability of primary prevention has been readily acknowledged, especially if the methods of treatment of overt disease have been less than adequate. When the "cause" of a disease was not known and it appeared to be related to the natural phenomena of aging, it has been difficult to arouse much enthusiasm for determining the precursors in apparently healthy persons.

It is now well recognized that "risk factors" can be identified in the development of many diseases that have no known cause. However, a number of physicians still question the usefulness of such knowledge in the absence of proof that changes in these factors are of value and in the absence of practicable means of making the necessary changes.

The Framingham Study, as it has become known, was undertaken to determine the risk factors for coronary heart disease and other atherosclerotic disorders. Reports of the findings, published periodically in various medical journals, have covered particular aspects of the study in some detail and are still useful for those seeking answers to specific questions. I have frequently been asked whether there was a publication that told the entire story of the Framingham Study—a narrative that, without being too detailed, would give the reader a reasonably complete knowledge of the overall project. Because of the apparent need for such a report of this long-term study as it reached the end of its productive life, I undertook the writing of this book.

The Framingham Study has not been associated with the name of any particular investigator, as has been true of numerous other research projects. This is appropriate in view of the many individuals who have participated in the conduct of the program. Nevertheless, effective long-term studies do require the personal interest of one or more people for prolonged periods of time. My own role, therefore, has been to preserve the continuity of the project, to maintain uniformity in assessment of disease incidence and population characteristics, and to encourage all those concerned with the program to carry it through to completion. Of particular importance has been the constant rekindling of interest on the part of the participants, without whom there would have been no study.

I recognize that success in endeavors such as this one is a relative term. It is essential to maintain adequate follow-up of the study population, or a project fails. And a program must elicit positive evidence to support the hypotheses under investigation or it is considered unsuccessful, no matter how well it may have been conducted. Fortunately we in Framingham have been able to satisfy both of these major requirements.

The Framingham Study will be recorded in medical history as one approach to the analysis of a chronic disease of unknown etiology. Its pattern could be followed with many other disorders, but the effort and expense of undertakings of this magnitude make comparable programs seem unlikely, at least in the immediate future.

PREFACE

The Framingham Study required the services and assistance of a large number of individuals. I am grateful to the many medical colleagues and other staff members who worked so hard over the years to keep track of the participants and encourage their ongoing interest in the study, and who collected and evaluated the emerging data. I particularly wish to thank Patricia McNamara and Rita Nickerson for their continuing help in providing the finished data for this book. And I am especially indebted to Elizabeth Hawes, who helped prepare the manuscript for submission and made many valuable suggestions to clarify the content. Her willingness to spend unlimited time, and her dedication to the completion of the project, were of inestimable aid.

The members of the advisory committee, who gave freely of their time and advice, are indicated below:

Edward F. Bland, M.D.	Associate Director Good Samaritan Hospital Boston, Massachusetts
Laurence B. Ellis, M.D.	Chief of Cardiology Boston City Hospital
James M. Faulkner, M.D.	Dean, Boston University School of Medicine
Burton E. Hamilton, M.D.	Chief of Cardiology Boston Lying-In Hospital
Hugh K. Leavell, M.D.	Professor of Public Health Practice Harvard School of Public Health
Samuel A. Levine, M.D.	Chief of Cardiology Peter Bent Brigham Hospital Boston, Massachusetts
Benedict F. Massell, M.D.	Associate Director Good Samaritan Hospital
Loren D. Moore, M.D.	First Assistant Commissioner Massachusetts Department of Public Health
Samuel H. Proger, M.D.	Chief of Cardiology Tufts New England Medical Center Boston, Massachusetts
David D. Rutstein, M.D.	Professor of Preventive Medicine Harvard Medical School
Robert W. Wilkins, M.D.	Professor of Medicine Boston University School of Medicine

PREFACE

Although it is impossible to list all the individuals involved in the study over 24 years, I should like to express my gratitude for their work and acknowledge that without their collective effort the present book would not exist.

The Framingham Study was admittedly expensive, and I am grateful to all those whose generous contributions supported our work. For a number of years the entire cost was borne by the National Heart Institute. Later the Boston University Medical Center took over the task of raising the necessary funds; the following are the agencies that participated:

Alcoa Foundation
American Life Insurance Company
Armour and Company
Berkshire Life Insurance Company
The Burroughs-Wellcome Fund
Carter-Wallace, Inc.
Clark Charitable Trust
Coatings Engineering Corporation
Concordia Foundation Trust
Confederation Life Insurance
  Company
Cuna Mutual-Cumis Insurance
  Societies
Cutter Foundation
Employers-Commercial Union
  Insurance
Geigy Pharmaceutical Company
Gulf Oil Foundation
Hamilton Management Corporation
Hartford Insurance Group
Hoechst Pharmaceutical Company
Home Life Insurance Company
IBM Corporation
Ives Laboratories
Kansas City Life Insurance Company
Charles A. King Trust
Lincoln National Life Insurance
  Company
Massengill Pharmaceutical Company

William May Company
Oscar Mayer Foundation
Mercantile & General Reinsurance
  Company
Metropolitan Life Insurance
  Company
Monarch Life Insurance Company
National Coffee Association
Newmont Mining Corporation
New York Life Insurance Company
North American Reassurance
  Company
Pan American Life Insurance
  Company
Patriot General Life Insurance
  Company
Paul Revere Life Insurance Company
A. C. Ratshesky Foundation
Searle Medidata
Security Mutual Life Insurance
  Company
Southwestern Life Insurance
  Company
Tobacco Research Institute
United Life & Accident Insurance
  Company
Upjohn Company
Wabash Life Insurance Company
Wisconsin Life Insurance Company

Finally, my thanks are extended to the Commonwealth Fund for enabling me to prepare this manuscript for publication.

Contents

The Framingham Study

Introduction

1

LIFE EXPECTANCY TODAY beyond the age of 40 is not much different from that of a century ago. The increased longevity compared to a hundred years ago has been achieved by the greatly improved prevention of infant and childhood diseases. With few exceptions, the population now lives well into adulthood. Life expectancy at birth is approximately 68 years for men and 75 for women (U.S. Dept. HEW, 1972). However, around these average values is a wide range of variability; many persons survive well into their 80s or 90s, still in a reasonably good state of physical and mental health.

This improvement in life expectancy is a remarkable achievement. In spite of air and water pollution, the automobile with its attendant high accidental death rate, radiation hazards, food additives, and all the other physical and psychical trauma of modern society, life expectancy at birth has gone steadily *up*, not down. Most people succumb eventually to what in the past has been considered degenerative disease—cancer and atherosclerosis.

The Impact of Medical Care

Our system of medical care is often extolled by one group for the life expectancy of our citizenry, yet blamed by another for being less than in certain other countries. It is unlikely, however, that medical care per se actually contributes importantly to life expectancy (Petersen, 1970). Dramatic medical and surgical "advances" are applicable to a relatively small portion of the population, and the alleged benefits are often grossly overstated. The impact of coronary care units, which have multiplied in the United States, may turn out to be negligible when measured against mortality from heart disease. Although a dramatic discovery by which the atherosclerotic process could be reversed is conceivable, the possibility is not great, especially in long-standing disease. Once scarring and calcification have developed, the disease may well be irreversible. Although a continuing search for methods of reversing the disease process is in order, a primary preventive approach may be more promising.

From a practical standpoint it is fallacious to imply that all medical problems can be solved by developing preventive measures. It simply is not likely that the diseases which affect the older members of our population can be *prevented* altogether. It is much more reasonable to hypothesize that the onset of these diseases can be *delayed*. Furthermore, any measures that prevent death or short-term illness (such as myocardial infarction or pneumonia) may enable the survivor to live into an older age bracket in which development of chronic illness is highly probable. Lengthy hospital or nursing-home care may then be required, with the result that lifetime medical care is markedly increased.

What is needed is a combined approach to all disease whereby we concentrate on prevention or delay in onset but also provide medical care for overt clinical disease, its complications, and any disabilities that may be incurred. The medical profession has been accused of concentration on treatment of disease to the exclusion of prevention. A review of medical history will show, however, that whenever practicable preventive approaches have been developed, physicians have adopted them. If we are to achieve such measures in the atherosclerotic diseases, we must first determine what characteristics of host and environment lead to the early appearance of these disorders. This was the motivation for the project that came to be known as the Framingham Study. We shall see how this study evolved and examine the occurrence of atherosclerotic disease in the population relative to a number of characteristics, many of which are modifiable in a favorable direction. It is our hope that from this knowledge practicable preventive measures may be elicited.

Epidemiologic studies may involve the investigation of a disease at any stage. Thus, clinical trials of the efficacy of a particular drug in preventing recurrence or progression of a disease are epidemiologic studies. Similarly, investigations of the prognosis following onset of a disease are basically epidemiologic. However, the major thrust of epidemiologic investigation has to do with factors that affect the original development of the disease. Knowledge from such studies is applicable to primary prevention of the disease—the major goal of medical research.

The word *epidemiology* usually suggests a study of epidemics —the prevalence or incidence of disease in excess of that customarily observed. Generally, an epidemiologist is not consulted unless the increase is substantial. In the case of a disease that is endemic to a given area, a certain controllable amount may be acceptable. (Needless to say, if there is less than the usual amount of a particular disease in a community, this will be a matter of concern neither to the health department nor to the practicing physician.)

Rather than being concerned solely with epidemics, epidemiology should involve the study of all factors relevant to the development of a disease. In this framework epidemiology becomes a study of the *natural history of disease*. It should attempt not only to determine the particular circumstances under which a disease develops or flourishes, but also those surrounding the *absence* of or *significant decrease* in prevalence or incidence of the disease. The objective of epidemiologic studies should therefore be to determine the natural history of a given disease and to explore the behavior of the disease, whether its rate has increased or decreased, and the possible factors that might explain such behavior. From this knowledge it should be possible to suggest changes that might be brought about in either the host or the environment or both which would prevent the disease altogether or modify it favorably—either to delay its onset or diminish its complications.

Epidemiology utilizes measurement of both the prevalence and the incidence of disease; prevalence refers to the amount of disease existing at a particular time, whereas incidence refers to the number of new cases developing within a given period of time. The *rates* of disease occurrence are the basic measurements to be used for comparison. Explanations are sought to account for any observed *differences*. Because the epidemiologist is concerned with the amount of disease found in particular populations, he needs the collaboration of his statistical colleagues to help in the design of the study and to plan the collection, processing, and analyzing of the data. The statistical methodology may be simple or quite complex.

Since the task of the epidemiologist is to count the number of cases of disease developing in the population under study, he must set up rigid criteria for what constitutes a "case," so that those subjects developing disease can be clearly separated from the remaining population. Early on, an estimate must be made of the number of subjects from the population selected who are expected to develop disease over a projected period of time. This number must be large enough so that when the time comes to analyze the various associated factors, the size of the group with disease will be adequate.

The close involvement of epidemiology with statistics has led many physicians to conclude that epidemiologic studies are "merely statistical" and not related to clinical medicine. This belief has been encouraged by the use of imprecise diagnostic categories and attempts to relate disease occurrence to a number of factors that may appear irrelevant to a physician faced with a need for more action-oriented information. The finding of an association between a given factor and the occurrence of any disease has little meaning in itself. If the relationship is one that fits what is known about the disease and has a logical explanation, it is worth exploring further regardless of the strength of the relationship. If, however, the relationship is very powerful, it deserves careful scrutiny even though the alleged relationship may be unexplained at the time.

Of utmost importance is the selection of characteristics of both host and environment that are worthy of investigation. It is clearly impossible to become concerned with every facet of human life. It becomes necessary at a practical level to confine the investigation to hypotheses that are reasonable. Search for relationship between possible factors and disease development done at random is not an exercise likely to warrant the effort. In the absence of good hypotheses the research effort should be directed first toward finding such hypotheses, despite the difficulties involved.

Relationships between disease development and host or environmental factors are almost never absolute. Everyone exposed to an infectious agent does not develop the infection. Even in highly susceptible populations only some persons become ill. The task of the epidemiologist, assisted by his statistical colleagues, is to determine to what degree an observed relationship may be the result of chance and at what point the relationship is sufficiently strong that it may well be involved in causality. *Cause*, a word epidemiologists prefer to avoid, to many people implies a factor without which the disease would not occur. If it were used with this connotation, a conclusion would be reached that the tubercle bacillus was the inevitable cause of tuberculosis or that lead paint was the usual cause of lead poisoning. In actuality, all persons exposed to the tubercle bacillus do not develop clinical tuberculosis, nor do all those exposed to lead paint develop lead poisoning. Other factors also may be causally related. Malnutrition or alcoholism may be responsible for the development of clinical tuberculosis following an exposure to tubercle bacilli, which under other circumstances would not have produced disease. Similarly, the presence of lead paint on a windowsill does not by itself produce lead poisoning; the factors that induce a child to chew the paint are obviously just as responsible.

In the absence of a sine qua non for disease development, the term *cause* becomes even more controversial. A combination of circumstances may lead to the increased occurrence of a disease, yet no single factor must necessarily be present. Although young male alcohol or drug addicts may contribute to a high rate of automobile accidents, clearly neither alcoholism nor drug addiction is necessarily the sole cause. Both of these conditions nevertheless are "causally" related, since youth, maleness, and the amount of alcohol or drugs used are importantly related to automobile accident rates. Thus we should speak of the *causes* of a disease rather than concentrating on a single cause. The task of the epidemiologist is to root out *all* the causes, all the various factors that act to increase the incidence of the disease. In addition, the relative importance of each of the factors involved must be assessed individually and in combination with other factors. On the basis of this information a rational explanation of pathogenesis and plans for control of the disease may be formulated.

Presentation of Epidemiologic Data

Reports from epidemiologic studies are usually presented in the form of the relative prevalence and/or incidence of the disease in populations that can be described and compared. Thus, if we wish to know whether the smoking of cigarettes contributes to the development of a particular disease, we must have comparable populations of persons smoking and not smoking cigarettes. We must determine the *rate* of occurrence of the disease in each of these populations. If a disease were nonfatal and left telltale evidence in those recovering, prevalence of the disease might be a satisfactory measurement. If, however, the mortality is high or recovery from the disease leaves no diagnostic stigmata, prevalence alone will not be an adequate index of the frequency of the disease. By determining incidence (that is, all the new cases that appear in a population previously free of the disease) we can be much more certain that our estimate is accurate. We are particularly helped in our study if some stigmata of the disease remain for an indefinite period, as with electrocardiographic evidence of myocardial infarction.

In order that the reader can make an unbiased interpretation, the actual findings themselves should be presented—perhaps as crude rates (the number of cases developing from the number of subjects studied). In order to permit easy comparison, the crude incidence data should be converted to rates based on populations of standard size (usually 1,000). Crude incidence rates give the probability that a disease will occur over a stated period of time in a population free of disease at the initiation of the study. However, these figures may give a distorted picture of the true incidence of the disease for persons who remain at risk. During the observation period a number of individuals will die accidentally, succumb to a different disease, or otherwise be lost to observation. In addition, those subjects who develop the disease early in the course of the observation period henceforth are no longer at risk of acquiring it. In any population with which we start, the number at risk constantly becomes smaller. By calculating this changing number of subjects and the time during which they are at risk, we obtain a corrected rate that answers the question of *potential* disease development if other factors do not intervene.

When young individuals are followed for only a brief time, the crude rate and the corrected rate will differ very little; the death rate is low and few people are lost to observation. In older subjects, however, especially if the observation period is a long one, the crude rate may greatly underestimate the risk, because of removal by death from some other disease of a large number who would have developed the disease in question had they remained under observation.

More sophisticated methods of calculating and expressing the relative probability of developing a disease are available. Physicians unfamiliar with statistical methodology are understandably confused by many complicated statistical expressions and accept the conclusions without questioning or understanding them. Insofar as possible the presentation of data and illustrative material in this volume will be in the simplest terms, so that those who have had limited exposure to statistical methodology will understand what they are reading.

Statistical Significance

If we are comparing the incidence of disease in two or more groups that differ in one or more characteristics (the importance of which we wish to evaluate), the meaning of the variations in the data, if any, should be indicated by determining the *statistical significance* of the differences. This figure, calculated from the actual observations, provides an index of the seriousness with which the findings should be considered. It tells the investigator in mathematical terms the probability that differences observed are the result of chance alone.

By convention, when a given set of observations could not occur by chance more frequently than one time in 20 ($p = 0.05$), such observations are usually accepted as statistically significant. Many observations that do not reach this level of probability may nevertheless turn out to be caused by other than chance. Furthermore, differences that are statistically significant at any level of probability could, after further data become available, turn out to be chance observations, especially if the

determination of significance is based on small numbers. Therefore it is highly desirable that any studies be repeated, preferably by other investigators. If subsequent work fails to confirm
the original findings, conclusions based on the earlier investigation must be questioned. On the other hand, if repeated studies
show similar relationships, it becomes impossible to disregard
the conclusions and their statistical significance is markedly
enhanced.

One distinction discussed infrequently but of great conse-
quence to practicing physicians is that between statistical significance and clinical importance. This may also involve what has
been referred to as "administrative significance" (Buncher,
1973). Observations on differences in many characteristics
(such as blood-pressure level or weight), if made on very large
numbers of subjects, may find small differences, which because
of the size of the population are highly significant statistically.
The physician may decide that regardless of the significance
level, the findings have no clinical importance; they do not warrant action. Public health officials will not find them administratively significant. This distinction is often difficult. For example, if two populations differed in average values of systolic
blood pressure by as little as 5 mm Hg, this difference might be
highly significant statistically. Few physicians would believe
that any causal hypothesis proposed to account for the difference had much to offer in terms of medical practice. Yet any
public health effort that caused the average blood pressure of
the population to drop by even this small amount might be reflected eventually by measurable differences in longevity or
morbidity from cardiovascular disease.

An epidemiologic study may be relatively crude or quite refined. The former includes such gross observations as report-
edly higher death rates from a given disease in one country than
in another, or comparison between reported fat consumption
and heart disease. These studies are often labeled "statistical,"
which implies only that they are based purely on reported statistics that can be obtained by any interested person. Examples
of more refined epidemiologic studies include carefully planned
clinical investigations in well-defined populations, and well-
designed clinical trials of the efficacy of drugs or surgical procedures. Physicians are understandably critical of studies that
attempt to reach conclusions about the etiology of disease by

demonstration of association between crude measures of disease prevalence or incidence and even cruder methods of determining a population characteristic. While recognizing the alleged association as an interesting observation, they wish to know more about the specific characteristics of those *individuals* who actually develop the disease in question and the validity of the assigned diagnosis.

Physicians are particularly familiar with the contributions of epidemiology in infectious diseases. The classic studies of Snow, and his demonstration of how an epidemic of cholera could be stopped by cutting off the water supply simply by removing the handle of the water pump, impressed on everyone the value of the epidemiologic approach (Snow, 1936). Those who have insisted on complete knowledge of the pathogenesis of a disease before tackling its control need to be reminded that the cholera vibrio was unknown at the time of Snow's monumental contribution. Observations of the time and place where the disease occurred and other circumstances, in this case the source of the water supply, were sufficient to pinpoint the major environmental factor related to the disease.

James Lind of the British Navy, as early as 1747, showed clearly that scurvy could be prevented by the administration of small amounts of lemon juice (Lind, 1953). His contribution led to the control of this disease many years before vitamin C was discovered.

In general, the shorter the incubation period—the time between apparent good health and the earliest manifestation of disease—the easier it is to conduct an epidemiologic study. If only a few days are required for fully developed disease to occur, it is not difficult to check various aspects of the life of subjects manifesting the disease and determine how they differ from those of subjects remaining free of disease. The longer the period of time, the more difficult the task becomes. In diseases such as atherosclerosis, which takes decades to develop, it is not surprising that the contributory factors have been so elusive.

*Problems in the Epidemiologic Study of
Atherosclerotic Disease*

The observations of Virchow (1856) concerning the changes in the arterial wall in atherosclerosis paved the way for intensive study of the pathology of this disease. Deposition of lipid material in the intima of the medium-sized and larger arteries eventually leads to an "atheromatous" deposit and ulceration of the intimal surface in contact with the circulating blood. The process is entirely asymptomatic and may take many years. It is not until the encroachment of the atheromatous material on the arterial lumen markedly interferes with the blood supply of the heart muscle, the brain, the lower extremities, or less frequently the kidney or other organs, that attention is called to the disorder. When the atheromatous lesion on the arterial wall ulcerates, destroying the integrity of the intimal surface, a nidus for clot formation is set up. Sudden clot formation may bring about complete ischemia and result in infarction of a segment of the heart muscle, brain, or other organ.

Because atherosclerotic disease can remain latent for so many years, and the clinical manifestations of its presence be delayed until well along in the course of atherosclerosis, epidemiologic study is extremely difficult. In fact, in the living it is usually not possible to study human atherosclerosis per se; rather, we must examine one or more of its clinical sequelae. This has caused some medical scientists to question the wisdom of attempting to study the epidemiology of atherosclerotic diseases until better methods are available for determining the presence of atherosclerotic changes and for quantitating the lesions with regard to both the surface area of the arterial walls involved and the degree of narrowing of the arterial lumen. By means of arteriography it is possible to make determinations of the degree of narrowing of the arterial lumen prior to the development of symptoms of ischemia. However, because of the invasive nature of such a test it is practicable and ethical only in the presence of symptoms suggestive of ischemia—and then only if a definitive procedure to relieve the ischemia is to be considered.

Some investigators have attempted to relate host and environmental factors to the pathological changes in the walls of sections of arteries removed surgically, such as aneurysms replaced by prostheses or arterial occlusions treated by bypass surgery. Unfortunately in this type of investigation the possible risk factors are evaluated very late in the course of the disease. In addition, the subjects studied are relatively older and comprise only the survivors of a much larger cohort, many of whom have died of the same disease at a younger age. Conclusions from such studies must be accepted with extreme caution. The characteristics of persons who already have advanced disease are not necessarily the same as those that predispose to the disease. The extreme emaciation observed in patients with advanced malignancy does not suggest that weight loss predisposes to cancer. Observations of population characteristics must be made well before disease becomes overt if the relation of these characteristics to the development of the disease is to be established with reasonable certainty.

The Framingham Study was undertaken with full knowledge of the difficulties of conducting long-term epidemiologic studies. It was recognized that there were specific problems related to studying atherosclerotic disease which, although beginning very early in life, did not present clinically until well into adulthood. Methods for detecting the clinical manifestations were available but imperfect; the degree to which they reflected the underlying atherosclerotic process was far from absolute. Several rational hypotheses had been proposed, but many others would undoubtedly be conceived too late for inclusion in the study.

The Framingham Study is properly considered an exercise in clinical epidemiology. The data were obtained solely from clinical evaluation of patients in a one-to-one relationship with a physician or other health worker. The major advantage of this study over many clinical investigations involving hospital or clinic populations is in the selection and follow-up of the study cohort, the uniformity of the clinical evaluation of the subjects, and the inclusion of both healthy and ailing subjects.

Faced with a series of obstacles that may be difficult to overcome, some investigators may take the attitude, "They said it couldn't be done, so I didn't try." Fortunately those who planned the Framingham investigation rejected such an attitude and decided to undertake this project with the expectation that useful information could be obtained even though the available methodology had not been perfected.

The major concern of public health workers prior to World War II was the control of infectious diseases that had previously been the major causes of morbidity and mortality. Improved sanitation had greatly decreased the diarrheal diseases. Considerable strides had been made in controlling tuberculosis and

pneumococcal pneumonia. With the introduction of penicillin
in 1942 a further dramatic change in lessening the prevalence
and incidence of infectious diseases took place.

At the end of World War II officials in the Public Health Service were confronted with a changing health situation in this
country. If further advances were to be made, clearly they
would be in the realm of noninfectious disease. Of these, cardiovascular disease and cancer constituted the overwhelming
majority, with disorders of the heart and blood vessels approximately twice as common as cancer. Prior to 1950 cardiovascular disease consisted in large part of the late effects of rheumatic
fever and syphilis, both of which appeared conquerable with
methods of prevention and therapeutic care already developed.
The major remaining disease about which little knowledge of
either prevention or treatment had been accumulated was
atherosclerosis and its resultant effects on the heart, brain, and
other organs.

As the other countries of the world recovered from World
War II, it became possible to make meaningful comparisons of
the reported prevalence of atherosclerotic diseases in diverse
populations throughout the world. Many of the data were relatively crude and inaccurate. Nevertheless, they did suggest that
stroke and coronary heart disease were not uniformly prevalent
in all countries. Even allowing for the serious discrepancies in
diagnostic acumen in various countries, the large differences reported suggested that factors other than accuracy of diagnosis
might be responsible. But nosologic variability clearly was an
obstacle to be overcome.

The World Health Organization, which had replaced the
Medical Division of the former League of Nations, began efforts
to standardize diagnostic criteria for disease and to collect data
on morbidity and mortality of cardiovascular disease from its
member nations. One of the foremost pioneers in the field of
cardiovascular epidemiology, and the person who was most
vigorous in projecting the idea that atherosclerotic disease, particularly coronary heart disease, was not an inevitable result of
the aging process but rather was related to environmental factors, was Ancel Keys of the University of Minnesota. His observations on the differences in reported coronary heart disease

INTRODUCTION

rates and the relation of these rates to the nutritional status of the populations involved (especially their intake of fat) were of great importance in promoting further investigation of factors responsible for the alleged differences in cardiovascular diseases (Keys, 1948, 1980).

Organization of the Framingham Study

2

THE LONG AND HONORABLE HISTORY of the U.S. Public Health Service dates back to the early days of the new nation. In 1798 a Marine Hospital Service was established by Act of Congress. This organization was responsible for the medical care of merchant seamen and for prevention of the introduction of disease into this country. Because of its concern with immigration, quarantine and customs control, the Marine Hospital Service was closely associated with the old Revenue Cutter Service (forerunner of the present U.S. Coast Guard). Both services were therefore under the administrative control of the Treasury Department.

As the duties of the Marine Hospital Service expanded to include many more duties concerned with public health, its name was changed to the U.S. Public Health Service. One of the divisions developed under this agency was the Hygienic Laboratory, later to become known as the National Institute of Health (NIH). With the reorganization of the federal bureaucracy under President Franklin D. Roosevelt, the Public Health Service was transferred into the newly organized Federal Security Agency.

In the Public Health Service, a Division of Chronic Disease had been established and programs developed in an attempt to determine to what degree cardiovascular disorders might be preventable and what practicable measures might be undertaken. The epidemiology of these diseases was of primary concern. Characteristic of some of the earlier investigations were those on the prevalence and incidence of diabetes mellitus in Oxford, Massachusetts (Wilkerson and Ford, 1949). Much of the stimulus behind these investigations came from Assistant Surgeon General Joseph Mountin. Among the various projects he considered of prime importance to the development of preventive measures in chronic disease was a long-term epidemiologic study of atherosclerotic cardiovascular disease.

Prior to World War II the NIH had been a relatively small organization, largely concerned with laboratory studies of disease of public health importance at that time. The contributions of its scientists had been many, including the noteworthy studies of Goldberger in pellagra (Terris, 1964). The expansion of the National Institute of Health over the past 30 years to its present status as a collection of institutes organized to concentrate study of the many diseases that affect our population has been phenomenal (Sherman, 1977). To the original NIH a special institute for cancer research was added, followed in 1949 by the creation of the National Heart Institute. Prior to its establishment many of the functions which it was to assume had been carried out to a limited degree by other divisions of the Public Health Service. Although for several years there had been some indication that an institute for the study of heart disease would eventually be established, Mountin did not choose to wait. Under his overall direction efforts were made to establish studies of the epidemiology and possible prevention of heart disease. Two of these were located near each other in Framingham and in Newton, Massachusetts. The emphasis of the Framingham Study was to be epidemiologic. In Newton, practical approaches to prevention were the primary concern (Kattwinkel et al., 1951). The initial interest of the Framingham Study was in the development and testing of methods for the early detection of heart disease, and the screening of apparently well populations to determine asymptomatic disease.

Before Framingham was selected as a site for the study, several other locations had been suggested. Largely through the efforts of Dr. David D. Rutstein of the Harvard Medical School, it was decided to establish the study in Framingham (Dawber, Kannel, and Lyell, 1963). At the time it was a small, self-contained community of approximately 28,000 inhabitants, 18 miles west of Boston. Most of the residents were employed locally in well-established business and manufacturing activities. Medical care was obtained from local physicians, utilizing two hospitals near the center of the town. A town-appointed health agent maintained surveillance of health activities in the town.

One of the most potent factors influencing the decision to locate the program in Framingham was the presence of a highly cooperative and well-informed medical profession. A group of these physicians and other interested townspeople agreed to assist in an attempt to involve as many of the residents as possible in the study. The general plan was to select a reasonably stable population of adults who would vary in the characteristics believed to be related to coronary heart disease. An initial examination of these subjects would be carried out to determine the presence of any stigmata of existing disease. Those subjects showing no such evidence would then be followed for a proposed period of 20 years, to determine which of them would eventually develop coronary heart disease. During the study period an effort would be made to characterize each of the subjects with regard to a number of bodily traits, life habits, or other factors which were believed to relate in any way to the eventual development of this disease.

Dr. Gilcin F. Meadors, a young Public Health Service officer, was charged with organizing the Framingham Study (Dawber, Meadors, and Moore, 1951). He began by accepting volunteers from the town with the objective of developing a sufficiently large population for a long-term study of the epidemiology of coronary heart disease.

When the National Heart Institute was established in 1949, it appeared advisable to place certain existing programs under its jurisdiction. The first director, Dr. Cassius J. Van Slyke, was a career officer in the Public Health Service with considerable experience in public health work, including epidemiology. He had been directly involved in the highly successful Public Health Service efforts to control syphilis spearheaded by former Surgeon General Thomas Parran. Van Slyke was thoroughly committed to the need for knowledge of the epidemiology of a disease if preventive measures were to be achieved. It was therefore quite understandable that he would ask for the transfer of the incipient Framingham Study to the National Heart Institute. Because of the guidelines that research into methods of prevention and control of disease were a function of the National Institutes of Health, and projects concerned with practicable control measures belonged elsewhere in the Public Health Service, Mountin agreed—although he was obviously reluctant to part with a study in which he had been so deeply interested.

With the transfer of the Framingham Study to the National Heart Institute, certain changes were made immediately. One of the most important was reconsideration of the selection of the population at risk. Felix Moore became director of biometrics for the new Heart Institute, and one of his first duties was to determine the Framingham Study population. After reviewing the existing study design, his conclusion was that the population should be more representative of the Framingham residents than would be the case if the study were based purely on volunteers. One of the objectives of the Framingham investigation was to determine the incidence of coronary heart disease by age and sex with sufficient reliability so that these figures might be applicable to other areas of the United States. In addition, the incidence rates determined should be useful for comparison with other geographic areas throughout the world. Since the sample would be small relative to the total U.S. population, there was an overriding need to describe it carefully. Accordingly, Moore drew up a sample population selected from the list of town residents. (Each town in Massachusetts publishes annually the names, addresses, ages, and occupations of its residents over age 18. This census greatly facilitates epidemiologic studies of the type planned in Framingham.)

The decision regarding the size of the population needed was clearly a difficult one, since Moore had only gross estimates of what the strength of these and other factors to be studied might be. For purposes of determining the size, age, and sex makeup of the study population, it was possible to arrive at estimates based on the reported mortality from coronary heart disease. More precisely, persons in this category included those who had symptoms of angina pectoris or who had suffered myocardial infarction. Also included were those who had died suddenly or who had died after development of an illness suggesting myocardial infarction.

Data on the relative occurrence of these various manifestations of coronary heart disease were not readily available. In 1949 it was also not apparent that some of the various clinical entities might behave quite differently with regard to certain of the associated factors to be studied. Accordingly, the all-inclusive clinical category of coronary heart disease seemed a logical choice. Based on the expected incidence, an estimate was made that approximately 5,000 to 6,000 adult men and women would be required as the population at risk. Over a 20-year period sufficient numbers of subjects with this disorder would emerge to permit study of the relationship of those important characteristics that might predispose to coronary heart disease. In 1949, of the population of 28,000, there were approximately 10,000 persons in the town of Framingham, aged 30 through 59 years. Moore felt that if two-thirds of these could be brought in for examination and followed over the projected 20 years, an adequate number of subjects to meet the above requirements would be available.

The original concept at Framingham included epidemiologic study of both coronary heart disease and hypertension. Since newly developing hypertension could not be studied in those who already had elevated blood pressure, it was decided to remove from the long-term follow-up all persons who already had evidence of this disorder. However, since blood-pressure level was considered a possible important factor in the development of coronary heart disease, a subsequent decision was made to keep all subjects in the study regardless of their blood-pressure findings. The expectation was that enough new cases of hypertension might appear to permit studying the incidence of high blood pressure per se.

The decision to study coronary heart disease as the end point required a definition of this entity. Discussion of this problem will be found in Chapter 6. With the change of direction of the Framingham Study late in 1949 and its transfer to the National Heart Institute, Meadors became involved in other public Health Service activities. Van Slyke, the director of the Heart Institute, asked if I would consider accepting responsibility for the conduct of the program. I had worked with him previously at the former Marine Hospital (now the U.S. Public Health Service Hospital) in Staten Island, New York, and knew that his promise to support me in the Framingham Study could be relied upon. Van Slyke did not underestimate the difficulties of conducting a long-term medical investigation. His own syphilis studies had made him fully cognizant of the problems involved in long-term follow-up of human populations. Research exactly comparable to that contemplated in Framingham had not, in fact, been carried out successfully; there was no experience on which to draw. After careful consideration of the need for a long-term commitment if the Framingham Study were to succeed, I agreed to become its director, a post that I held for the next 16 years, followed by continued close association for a total of 30 years.

One notable study of cardiovascular disease had been attempted by Sir James Mackenzie in Scotland, who had considered the advisability of a long-term investigation in his own medical practice as early as 1921 (Mackenzie, 1926). Such a project appeared quite feasible in Great Britain and certain European countries because of the lack of mobility of the population, most of whom received medical care in the immediate vicinity, often from only one physician. The ability of practicing physicians to be simultaneously amateur epidemiologists has been attested to many times. Mackenzie, however, found the task he had set himself too difficult and was forced to abandon it. His efforts were not entirely wasted because a young American physician, the late Paul Dudley White, had spent some time with him and had learned to share his enthusiasm for a population study of cardiovascular disease. White's exposure to Mackenzie was undoubtedly responsible for his later practice of keeping careful and detailed records on his own patients and using these data to reach valuable conclusions regarding cardiovascular diseases. He was particularly concerned with the relative occurrence of these diseases in his practice and with the significance of many symptoms and signs in the diagnostic process.

As adviser to Van Slyke at the Heart Institute, White showed a particular interest in the Framingham Study, of which he was one of the major supporters. Not everyone at the institute concerned with the direction of cardiovascular disease research was committed to the value of epidemiologic studies: many physicians and other investigators then, as now, believed that the answer to most of the important questions regarding the natural history of atherosclerotic vascular disease would come from basic laboratory research, not from study of the disease in man. That physicians of the caliber of White so strongly endorsed this investigation was therefore of great importance.

From the town census list the residents were categorized according to family size: one-member families, two-member families, three-member families, and those with four or more in the family. Lists of each of these family groups were arranged alphabetically and every third family was eliminated. The result was a list of 6,507 individuals—the population to be invited for examination. Those subjects free of disease at the initial examination would constitute the population to be followed. The expectation was that almost all the selected subjects would respond to the invitation to an initial examination.

The subjects were advised of the long-term character of the study and the need to return for reexamination at two-year intervals. This schedule was proposed because it would take two years to examine the entire population. In addition, the time period was believed short enough that no serious interim illness would be overlooked.

A health educator joined the study and proceeded to set up a community organization to encourage the selected subjects to come in. Volunteers were accepted for examination and in turn were asked to approach a number of persons on the selected list to obtain their participation. As a result, 68.6 percent of the selected subjects eventually came into the new medical clinic. The derivation of the Framingham Study population is summarized in Table 2-1. Much thought and effort went into further efforts to enlist the remaining 31.4 percent who did not participate. The results of this effort were essentially nil. The reasons given for nonparticipation, as recorded by the recruitment volunteers, included religious persuasion, receipt of medical care from a personal physician, and unwillingness to spend the time required (Dawber, Kannel, and Lyell, 1963). My own feeling is that the reasons given were largely those which the subjects believed would be acceptable to the staff of the study. I concluded from personally interviewing a sample of the nonparticipants that fear of what might be found upon examination was the major reason for noninvolvement. This problem is of considerable interest to anyone who plans to undertake a similar general

Table 2-1 Derivation of the Framingham Study population.

	No. men	No. women	Total
Random sample	3,074	3,433	6,507
Respondents	2,024	2,445	4,469
Volunteers	312	428	740
Respondents free of CHD[a]	1,975	2,418	4,393
Volunteers free of CHD	307	427	734
Total free of CHD: the Framingham Study group	2,282	2,845	5,127

[a]CHD = coronary heart disease.

population study or become in any way involved in the delivery of medical care. The assumption of many physicians that the people whom they might have occasion to serve are willing, and in fact anxious, to place themselves under medical surveillance was not verified by the Framingham Study.

Many of those involved in the conduct of the study were greatly concerned about the lack of total participation by those who had been selected. The extent to which generalizations might be made on the basis of a random sample could be greatly diminished by the limited response of the selected participants. However, figures on the prevalence of disease in this population, although desirable, were a minor objective. The degree to which the incidence figures might be biased was not clear. The major effect of the lack of total participation was to reduce the variability of some of the factors studied. Thus, a higher percentage of single males, excessive users of alcohol, and subjects with lower educational attainment failed to participate than would have been expected if the response had been strictly random.

Many epidemiologists become overly concerned about the degree to which a sample is representative of a larger population. In many ways the efforts to obtain complete participation of the entire selected sample were not justified. The objectives of the Framingham Study did include determination of the absolute incidence of the various manifestations of atherosclerotic disease. Yet the determination had only limited applicability, since the population of this New England town was in itself not totally representative of the United States. There were virtually no blacks or Orientals, and the composition of the white population was not necessarily that of white populations elsewhere.

Random sampling is not essential if the purpose of an epidemiologic study is to compare subgroups of the population determined by specific characteristics. The primary concern should be that the population contain sufficient numbers of subjects with these characteristics to enable comparison. Selected samples may be perfectly satisfactory to study the effect of such factors as varying blood-pressure level on disease outcome. The only requirement is that the sample contain adequate numbers of subjects in the different blood-pressure categories.

The problem of obtaining patient participation is important to anyone who practices medicine or has occasion to observe subjects in an ongoing medical study. The initial approach fails to recruit those individuals who are "loners," who have personality defects, or who are prejudiced against participation in medical projects. Initially, those who report for examination are willing participants. However, they range from enthusiastic volunteers to very reluctant persons who may have been "dragged" to the physician by a spouse or friend. The former will continue to participate unless some untoward, unpleasant experience "turns them off." The latter may need to be recruited anew at each attempt to maintain contact.

From the very first, I believed that the continued participation of our study population would depend almost entirely on the treatment they received at the time of each examination. In studies in which the follow-up consists largely in obtaining information about the subject, not requiring his presence, this problem is minimal. In the Framingham Study it was absolutely necessary that the subject return again and again for reevaluation, since the end point was not only death but clinical disease requiring personal examination. Plans were made to procure pertinent medical data on all subjects from other sources as well. This information served a three-fold purpose: (1) to help determine the cause of death; (2) to supplant the clinical examination in subjects who were not available; and (3) to supplement information gathered at the biennial examinations.

The receptionist contacted each of the subjects in turn through family groups and tried to make an appointment for examination within the next few weeks. This often required repeated phone calls, letters, and sometimes a personal visit. On completion of the examination the receptionist reiterated the need for biennial examinations and prepared the subjects for a renewed invitation two years hence.

All members of the staff were frequently reminded of the importance of the continued participation of those enrolled in the program, and that the conduct of each examination must be such that the subjects would be willing and even anxious to return for subsequent visits. Physicians, accustomed to seeing patients with problems they wish to discuss, are inclined to believe that anyone is willing to wait in the reception room indefinitely in order to be examined. Nothing could be further from the truth when the evaluation of apparently healthy and asymptomatic individuals is undertaken. Such persons have limited interest in medical attention unless some specific objective can be made clear.

Although the concept of health maintenance is gradually becoming more generally understood, it is still far from being totally accepted. When the Framingham Study was organized, the concept was relatively new. Even among the medical profession there was considerable skepticism about the benefit of screening procedures and periodic examinations. This skepticism still remains. One very helpful factor in the recruitment of subjects was the relatively strong endorsement of the physicians practicing in the Framingham area. Although there has been increasing mistrust of the medical profession as a whole, it is remarkable that most patients exempt their own physician from the criticism they level so readily against the profession. The confidence of the Framingham subjects in their family physicians motivated them to ask their advice regarding participation in the study. In almost every instance they received the reassurance they sought.

Initial Examination of the Framingham Population

With few physical changes and little expenditure of money, a reasonably efficient clinic and laboratory were established at the Framingham Union Hospital, where readily identifiable

space was allocated to the study. Initial examinations were be-
gun in the spring of 1950. As expected, some of the original volunteers fell into the selected sample and thus had been seen
already.

In the evaluation of the population the major problems centered on the depth of the interview and examination. A number
of hypotheses had been proposed that called for information
obtained by interview, examination, and laboratory studies.
The time well people will devote to their medical evaluation
when it is not directly concerned with an immediate medical
problem is limited. Invasive procedures may be neither feasible
nor ethical. Definite constraints of time, practicability, and
ethics require that any evaluation of subjects in the type of epidemiologic study proposed be modified over what many physicians might wish to conduct on their own patients. In view of
these constraints, the initial examination was concerned primarily with determination of a disease-free population and collection of data characterizing the population with regard to the
major hypotheses proposed. Testing of other hypotheses was
deferred for later examinations, when adequate time could be
allotted and a satisfactory evaluation made.

Follow-Up in the Framingham Study

Since participation by the selected random sample of subjects
in the study was less than anticipated, we decided to include
some of the volunteers who had not been selected for the original cohort. The 740 subjects who were added were kept in a
special category, since as volunteers their characteristics might
be somewhat different from the selected group (see Table 2-1).
Later experience failed to indicate any important differences, so
their inclusion in the study population was eventually justified.

As indicated previously, the selection of a completely representative sample is essential if the objective is to generalize from
data on the prevalence or incidence rate of a disease to a much
larger population. If, however, the ultimate objective is to compare subgroups of the population with regard to various characteristics, the need to obtain a completely random representative population, although still desirable, is much less. Strictly
speaking, the study population in Framingham was made up
completely of volunteers, in that the final decision to participate

or not was their own. While their degree of enthusiasm varied considerably, they did not constitute a captive population. At each successive examination there were many subjects who did not report (for a number of reasons), yet the nonrespondents did not represent the same subjects at each biennial visit. The result was an overall loss to follow-up of only 2 percent.

At each of the biennial visits a medical history, physical examination, blood studies, and other laboratory work were completed. Any symptoms of illnesses that had developed since the previous visit were reviewed. Interim hospitalization or medical visits were recorded. All these data were carefully collected and collated by the Framingham staff under the direction of a statistician, who worked with a committee of three physicians to review all pertinent medical information. Included were death certificates, medical examiners' and coroners' reports, statements of personal physicians, and other facts concerning the circumstances surrounding death (which often required additional information beyond the formal report). Reports of hospitalization were obtained and any autopsy findings reviewed. Since the autopsy rate in most U.S. communities is relatively low (approximately 30 percent in Framingham), the use of such data for diagnostic purposes is limited. Here they were used for confirmation only.

Electrocardiograms, recorded both in our clinic and elsewhere, were reviewed individually as well as compared with all others obtained on a given subject. This procedure was particularly valuable in that it elucidated changes that were diagnostic, even though the individual electrocardiograms without comparative evaluation might be classified as within normal limits or nondiagnostic of specific pathology. It also demonstrated that some subjects who generated electrocardiographic tracings suggesting previous myocardial infarctions had in fact maintained such patterns for years (particularly the Q_2, Q_3, Q_{AVF} pattern). The committee of physicians had the responsibility of putting together all the data available on each subject at every biennial examination and classifying the individual according to the end points of disease. A neurologist participated in all decisions relating to cerebral vascular disease.

Because of the limited time allotted to each medical visit, the content of the initial examination was curtailed. Certain important hypotheses were to be tested at later visits, including the relationship of physical activity, dietary intake, and emotional and psychic stress. One reason for postponing the testing of such hypotheses was the obvious difficulty of measuring the variables involved. Methods of assessment of normal physical activity, food intake, and particularly the degree of stress to which an individual is exposed were not available and still are the subject of controversy. The accuracy with which categories of each of these variables can be distinguished is not established, since there is no absolute measurement against which any method can be tested. After exploring possible methods of collecting data on several additional variables, we included them in subsequent examinations with full knowledge of the limitations of the methodology.

Compilation of Data

The data collected on the subjects at each examination were recorded on self-coding forms, then transferred directly to punch cards and later to tapes for computer analysis. All other material was prepared similarly for analytical study.

In the early part of an epidemiologic study there is a fairly long period during which the major task is that of collecting data in routine fashion. Since the subjects in whom there is major interest for incidence purposes must necessarily be initially free of disease, the effort at first is directed toward identifying all persons with any clinical evidence of the disease under study. To young physicians trained in medical diagnosis and anxious to test their skills in the therapeutic field, the examination of apparently healthy individuals is not exactly a rewarding task. Fortunately the Framingham Study was able to recruit for short periods of time young physicians who had completed their training in medicine and cardiology and volunteered for duty in the Public Health Service. As might be expected, such physicians tended to look at each subject as a potential patient —someone with a disease. There was a tendency to interpret any symptoms as indicative of pathology. This was desirable in obtaining a study population free of disease, but needed careful control later on when new "cases" of disease developed in the previously well population.

As the study progressed and the population was brought

back for reexamination at two-year intervals, increasing numbers of participants were removed from the disease-free category and classified under the various rubrics of atherosclerotic disease. Not until seven years after the initiation of the study was a sufficient number of subjects classified as having developed coronary heart disease to permit even a preliminary report of the findings (Dawber, Moore, and Mann, 1957). Strongly suggestive evidence that some of the hypotheses under study would be supported by the data was already available from the work of others and from the impressions of the clinicians on the advisory committee. The first report of the Framingham findings to confirm these impressions kindled the enthusiasm of the staff and encouraged a search for additional hypotheses to be investigated.

The original plan envisioned a 20-year study. As time went by and increasing numbers of subjects developed disease so that more definitive testing of the several hypotheses was possible, we wondered how long to continue our surveillance of the population. In any long-term research the point beyond which the collection of additional information is no longer worthwhile is difficult to determine (Cohen, 1977). With each successive reevaluation the increased numbers of subjects in the various disease categories permitted more in-depth analysis of the factors under investigation. This, in turn, led to interest in the study of many questions not originally anticipated, but which would require a still larger population for meaningful analysis and therefore a need to continue the program. As might be expected, differences of opinion were voiced regarding the merits of following this population indefinitely. Even before the 20-year point had been reached, extramural committees were appointed to review the progress of the Framingham Study and to advise the National Heart Institute regarding the wisdom of continuing the program as originally established. By 1970, after 20 years of operation, a review committee recommended that clinical examinations be discontinued, inasmuch as the major hypotheses had been adequately tested. This decision was not approved by many persons, both inside and outside the National Institutes of Health. The Heart Institute indicated that it would follow the recommendations of the review committee. Some who disagreed tried to have the decision reversed. Since this was not successful, the suggestion was made to me that there should be an attempt to obtain funds from other sources to continue the study under private auspices. Accordingly, through the sponsorship of the Boston University Medical Center, a campaign was launched to finance an additional 5-year period of follow-up and evaluation of the Framingham population. Thanks to the support of a number of foundations, industrial enterprises, insurance companies and private individuals, it became possible to continue the study without interruption for another 4 years (2 cycles) and to complete 24 years of follow-up, which serves as the basis for the present report.

Upon completion of this phase of the study in 1975, the National Heart, Lung, and Blood Institute reassessed its former decision and supported a follow-up of the population through a contract to Boston University Medical Center. The collection of additional data on stroke, peripheral artery disease, and certain noncardiovascular diseases has been made possible by the extra years of follow-up. From the continuing observation of the Framingham population it may still be possible to add to our knowledge of the natural history of cardiovascular and other diseases in the aging population.

In the course of the study I was frequently approached by investigators, both within and without the National Institutes of Health, who wished to test one or another hypothesis. If these required access to a large human population which was already available and well described, it was only natural that the population laboratory at Framingham would be considered suitable. Fortunately a decision had been made not to permit any interference with the main objective of this study—delineation of cardiovascular disease. From time to time an investigator would suggest inclusion in the protocol of a pet hypothesis regarding atherosclerotic disease. Where practicable, we obliged—if careful review indicated the task to be worth the effort.

At one period of our work there was great interest in the development and maintenance of population laboratories, of which Framingham might be considered a prototype. The objective of these units was to provide an established pool of subjects in which new hypotheses could be tested. The concept had many things to recommend it. The cost of obtaining, organizing, and maintaining contact with populations the size of the Framingham Study is not inconsiderable. Without specific hypotheses that have important implications for human health, maintenance of population laboratories has not appeared feasible. We frequently considered the possibility of conducting studies other than those for which the population was derived. A few actually were successfully undertaken (Friedman, Kannel, and Dawber, 1966; Vander, Gaston, and Dawber, 1968). A major contribution was research on the study of eye diseases, conducted through the sponsorship of the National Eye Institute. Some reports on this work have been published and more are in preparation (for example, Kahn et al., 1977). Senile mental deterioration is currently being investigated.

Because of the location of the Biometrics Division of the National Institutes of Health in Bethesda, Maryland, and the availability of the NIH computer facilities, data analysis was conducted in Bethesda rather than at the Framingham locale under the direct supervision of the investigators. Computer technology at the time was still not well advanced and it seemed advisable to acquiesce to this arrangement. However, the decision presented many difficulties. The separation of the investigators collecting the data from those directly responsible for its analysis became a real problem. In spite of frequent meetings of all concerned, I found that as principal investigator I had less and less control over the analysis. In addition, the staff at the National Institutes of Health became increasingly possessive of the data, ostensibly to preserve the confidentiality of medical records. The matter came to a head when the task of continuing the examination was assumed by the Boston University group under my direction. The question of ownership of the data still has not been completely resolved and has arisen in other studies financially supported by the NIH.

My own insistence was that the data collected by an investigator in a study under his personal direction are primarily his. They must be available to him for analysis and reporting. The National Heart, Lung, and Blood Institute authorities took the view that the data were theirs and were not to be released to anyone. Fortunately, we arrived at reasonably amicable arrangements whereby earlier data were made available to me. The lesson I learned was that under no circumstances should any scientific investigator allow his work to be controlled by others who act not strictly as coinvestigators but as analysts of the findings of the research.

Diagnostic Categories of Atherosclerotic Disease

3

THE FIRST OBJECTIVE of an epidemiologic study is to determine the prevalence and incidence of the disease under study. To obtain these data, which can be expressed according to age and sex as the most obvious and easily measurable variables, the investigator must be able to recognize the various clinical manifestations of the disease. Furthermore, he must describe them in sufficient detail that others can, if desired, repeat the study with assurance that all concerned are referring to the same disease entity. This philosophy may seem elementary to physicians accustomed to making clinical diagnoses in everyday medical practice. However, if the physician analyzes his thought processes in arriving at a clinical diagnosis, he soon realizes that many of the factors that enter into his decision making are poorly defined. The diagnosis he arrives at is—or should be—based on the best interests of the patient. These interests are not identical with those of a research study. The practitioner's conclusions may involve *over*diagnosis if the objective is to bring under careful surveillance all those with a possibly severe illness or contagious disease, or they may call for playing down the symptomatology if anxiety appears to be the major problem. A working diagnosis of myocardial infarction, for example, may be made by a concerned practitioner and possibly adhered to, even though all the elements of such a diagnosis for scientific purposes may not be present.

Many times the clinician may feel certain that the patient has had a small cerebral infarction despite the fact that objective evidence of such an event may not be obtainable. Changes in the patient's personality or behavior, often impossible to measure, may lead the physician to conclude that organic changes in the patient's cerebrum have occurred. Physicians are frequently disturbed by the unwillingness of medical researchers to accept clinical impressions and instead to insist on objective evidence; they fail to appreciate that both are of value, depending on the purpose for which they are to be used.

Epidemiologic studies based upon diagnostic data obtained by a number of physicians who have no common agreement on the diagnostic criteria must be accepted with reservation. Death certificates are commonly utilized in determining the clinical diagnosis of cause of death. Unfortunately, there are no strict criteria to guide the physician completing the death certificate, even if he were willing to follow them. Anyone familiar with the various factors that enter into the preparation of death certificates recognizes the pitfalls of total reliance on the information so provided. In many diseases additional information must be obtained and corroborated before the cause of death can be ascertained (Moriyama, 1964; Moriyama, Dawber, and Kannel, 1966).

In the study of mortality from malignant disease, death certificates have proved quite reliable, since in our society it is highly unlikely that anyone dying of cancer will not have been under medical attention. If that medical care has been reasonably competent, a diagnosis will have been made and verified by laboratory studies early in the course of the disease. On the other hand, death in an apparently healthy person or in anyone who has not been under medical surveillance may have many different causes. The judgment of the certifying physician becomes crucial and determines the reported cause of death, often when there is no other objective data upon which to rely.

The epidemiologist wishes to establish diagnostic categories that are easily definable. The definitions of disease categories should be based upon information that is readily available from procedures that are practicable and accessible to the large majority of those called upon to diagnose the disease. The criteria for diagnosis should be specific. It is with regard to these criteria that the epidemiologist differs most from the physician in clinical practice. The physician must include all possible suspects to ensure that no one with a disease has been overlooked, knowing full well that many may not in fact have the disease. The eventual intent of the epidemiologist, on the other hand, is to compare the characteristics of those who develop disease with those who do not. The former group is almost always quite small and should contain as few persons as possible who do not have the disease. If the small "diseased" cohort is too diluted by the inclusion of a number of subjects without the disease, a relationship to some predisposing factor may be so minimized as to be lost. On the other hand, the inclusion of a relatively small number of subjects with disease (or possible disease) will not seriously affect characterization of the large nondiseased group.

The major organs affected by atherosclerotic disease are the heart, the brain, and the lower extremities. These three categories constitute the disorders that have been studied in Framingham. Definitions of clinical entities will therefore be confined to them. Less frequently, impaired blood supply resulting from atherosclerosis may produce clinical evidence of renal disease, intestinal disease, endocrine impairment, or other systemic disorder. The relative importance of the major clinical manifestations of atherosclerotic disease may be assessed from the observations of 24 years in the Framingham Study (Table 3-1).

Coronary Heart Disease

The heart muscle is primarily dependent on the coronary arteries for its blood supply. Some endocardial tissue may receive support directly from the blood in the atria and ventricles, but this must be minimal. Adequate function of the heart muscle requires patent coronary arteries which can supply a sufficient amount of blood while the individual is at rest and at whatever level of activity he may be called upon to perform.

As atheromatous plaques build up on the intimal wall, the lumen of the vessel involved decreases. With some increase in velocity of the blood in the region of constriction a normal

DIAGNOSTIC CATEGORIES OF ATHEROSCLEROTIC DISEASE

Table 3-1 Clinical manifestations of atherosclerotic disease. The data show the number of cases that developed over 24 years from the original population of 5,127.

No. of subjects who developed—	Men	Women
Coronary heart disease		
Angina pectoris	277	243
Total myocardial infarction	365	155
Myocardial infarction by electrocardiogram	301	121
Coronary insufficiency	71	53
Sudden death	130	43
Death, not sudden	150	75
Stroke		
Atherothrombotic brain infarction	94	105
Intracerebral hemorrhage	9	7
Subarachnoid hemorrhage	15	20
Cerebral embolism	23	25
Peripheral arterial disease		
Intermittent claudication	155	103
Congestive heart failure	181	156

blood flow may be maintained. Because of this, and some reserve beyond absolute need, the coronary arteries may continue to supply adequate blood to the myocardium even after considerable narrowing of the lumen has taken place even in the presence of advanced atherosclerosis. Eventually, however, the atheromatous encroachment on the lumen of the coronary artery reaches a point such that when a greater demand for oxygen is made by the myocardium than can be supplied, myocardial ischemia takes place.

Some prefer to use the term *ischemic heart disease* to indicate that the changes in the myocardium and the resulting psysiologic, functional, and pathological changes are caused by ischemia. Since, for practical purposes, myocardial ischemia is almost always the result of atherosclerotic disease of the coronary arteries, coronary heart disease becomes in effect synonymous with ischemic heart disease. However, it must be remembered that there are conditions other than coronary artery atherosclerosis that may result in myocardial ischemia. Severe anemia theoretically could do so. In reality, when evidence of myocardial ischemia is observed in the presence of anemia, the latter is almost always a compounding problem to narrowing of the coronary artery. A practical step the physician can take when he evaluates a patient with evidence of myocardial ischemia is, of course, to make sure that any anemia is corrected.

Infection with the spirochete of syphilis often damages the aortic wall. One pathological change is narrowing of the coronary ostia, which results in myocardial ischemia even in the absence of any significant degree of coronary atherosclerosis. Frequently syphilis and atherosclerosis occur together. The marked drop in the percentage of the population developing syphilis, the early detection of such infection, and its adequate treatment with penicillin have almost abolished newly developing cardiovascular syphilis. The extremely low rate of this disease in the Framingham population eliminated what might have been a real difficulty.

Rheumatic heart disease with damage to the aortic valve, both by producing regurgitation and/or stenosis, can impair coronary blood flow with resultant ischemia of the myocardium entirely unrelated to the atherosclerotic process. In 1950 the relatively high incidence of rheumatic fever in any New England population would have posed a problem in the study of ischemic heart disease except that subjects with rheumatic heart disease were identifiable. The Framingham Study has repeatedly sought to single out such patients in order that they be excluded from the atherosclerotic disease categories (Stokes and Dawber, 1956). The effect of this procedure would be to remove some subjects from the atherosclerotic coronary artery disease category where symptoms were the result of both disorders. Subjects demonstrating evidence of aortic stenosis were included in the rheumatic heart disease category even though it was recognized that many of them may have had calcific aortic stenosis of nonrheumatic etiology.

Because disease resulting from other than atherosclerosis can produce ischemia, the term *coronary heart disease* seems preferable to *ischemic heart disease* in reference to cardiac disorders resulting from atherosclerosis of the coronary artery. Some may prefer to speak of atherosclerotic coronary heart disease, to emphasize the basic disorder.

Clinical Manifestations

Atherosclerotic changes in the coronary artery can involve a large part of the surface area without producing any important change in the coronary blood flow if the plaques do not encroach on the coronary arterial lumen. On the other hand, a relatively small amount of the arterial wall may be involved by a plaque that builds up to encroach on the lumen and thus markedly impairs coronary flow with resultant myocardial ischemia. Because of these differences in behavior of the atherosclerotic process, there is often a discrepancy between the amount of arterial wall involved by atherosclerosis and the clinical manifestations of the disease. However, as might be expected, there is reasonably good correlation between the surface area involved and the degree of patency of the arterial lumen.

Undoubtedly the dynamics of blood flow play an important role. At autopsy, widespread damage to the intima of the aorta by atherosclerosis is commonly observed. In spite of this, negligible encroachment on the lumen of the aorta has occurred. Presumably any build-up or superimposed clot would be rapidly swept away by the forceful thrust of the blood column in the aorta. This may happen frequently in the carotid arteries, but is much less likely in the coronary arteries. As the lumen of the coronary arteries becomes narrowed, a point may eventually be reached at which the blood flow, although adequate when the subject is at rest, becomes insufficient to supply the oxygen demands of the myocardium at some level of work. This level will be variable but will be one that produces a rise in pulse rate and cardiac output. Some of the myocardium then becomes relatively ischemic. When the ischemia increases to a sufficient degree, the subject becomes aware of a definite feeling of discomfort—usually in the substernal area, frequently in the upper epigastrium, often radiating to the neck and down one or both arms.

Angina Pectoris

The term *angina pectoris*, originated by William Heberden as long ago as 1768 (Heberden, 1802), implies a choking sensation. Actually most patients describe a dull, heavy discomfort deep in the substernal area. The sensation is frequently linked in the patient's mind to the upper gastrointestinal system. Indigestion, often relieved by belching, may be noted. Symptoms typically are observed after a meal, particularly a heavy, fat-containing meal with slow emptying of the stomach. Slight exertion on a full stomach may be accompanied by anginal distress. The characteristics of the anginal syndrome are appearance of the symptoms *only* with exertion, excitement, or emotional distress and an ensuing *rise in pulse rate* related to an increase in the cardiac output. The disappearance of the anginal symptoms with the discontinuance of the exertion or other inciting factor, with a consequent drop in the pulse rate, is equally significant. Relief following the administration of nitroglycerin is also an important diagnostic clue. Angina pectoris is thus a *subjective* sensation, which can be described by the patient but which frequently requires considerable probing by the physician before a complete description can be obtained.

Chest discomfort is a rather frequent symptom, although all such pain, even in the suspicious substernal area, is not angina. The physician is often at a loss to know the derivation of the chest discomfort; it is frequently easier to conclude what it does *not* result from than to be certain of the cause. The relation to exertion or other factors that may significantly increase the pulse rate, and the disappearance when these inciting factors are removed, are the major elements in the diagnosis of angina. Since most patients learn rapidly what types of activity or environment bring on their discomfort and avoid such exposure, they may have long periods of freedom from symptoms. This "disappearance" of the disease may lead the physician to conclude that his diagnosis was in error, or that his therapy has been curative, only to have the symptoms return or some more serious manifestation of coronary disease appear.

Categories of clinical disease based on symptoms are not the best for epidemiologic purposes. Objective means of making a diagnosis of transient myocardial ischemia would be highly desirable. This has been attempted by obtaining electrocardiograms both at rest and with exercise. Such efforts, although partially successful, have definite limitations. Major interest has focused on the electrocardiogram.

The Electrocardiogram in Angina Pectoris

Patients with angina pectoris have short episodes of myocardial ischemia. If the ischemia is not too severe or prolonged, the myocardium is not damaged and the ischemic cells return to their former state: *there is no permanent myocardial disease.* In such individuals the resting electrocardiogram may be perfectly normal and unchanged from that recorded prior to the development of any anginal symptoms.

If the ischemia persists, some transient changes may develop that are reasonably characteristic. Electrocardiograms obtained before, during, and immediately following regulated exercise on a treadmill or by walking over steps, as in the Master's test, will detect these ischemic changes. While this test has become increasingly popular, it is not without hazards, it is time-consuming, and it has not always been practicable. Furthermore, angina pectoris is by definition a subjective sensation, which only the patient can describe. If chest discomfort is observed concomitantly with the development of ischemic electrocardiographic changes, the physician may feel more sure of his diagnosis. If, however, the electrocardiographic changes occur in the absence of any chest discomfort, the patient cannot be said to have angina pectoris but rather must be classified as having ischemic electrocardiographic changes with exercise.

As might be expected, the subject with recurrent symptoms of angina pectoris may well have had sufficient myocardial ischemia that permanent damage to some of the myocardial cells has resulted. In fact, the resting electrocardiograms of patients with a clinical diagnosis of angina have a greater degree of nonspecific abnormalities than is found in the general population. This figure is frequently estimated to be as high as 50 percent (Higgins, Kannel, and Dawber, 1965). Since these same changes are found in the nonanginal population, they cannot be used for diagnostic purposes in any absolute way.

Questionnaires for Angina Pectoris

Because of the difficulty in establishing a diagnosis of angina pectoris in a standardized manner, attempts have been made to use a uniform questionnaire and thus arbitrarily to determine the diagnosis. This attempt to change a subjective determination into an objective one, although considered laudable in many epidemiologic circles, is criticized by clinicians whose training in the art of history taking appears to be discounted.

Experience with questionnaires (such as that of Rose) has been reasonably satisfactory when applied to large populations

(Rose, 1965). The form was not intended as a tool for making the diagnosis in clinical practice but rather to detect disease in apparently well populations. In clinical epidemiology, where the determination of a case should be as accurate as possible without resorting to sophisticated procedures, there is still no substitute for a detailed medical history obtained by a physician completely familiar with the various manifestations of angina pectoris. The employment of standardized questionnaires in addition to such history taking is quite appropriate, but the substitution of a questionnaire for the more detailed probing methods of eliciting symptoms is not warranted.

At the time the Framingham Study was instituted there were no acceptable questionnaires. Most of the advisers to this study were clinically trained physicians who encouraged the use of acceptable clinical methods in diagnosis. Accordingly, all diagnoses of angina pectoris in this study represent the conclusions of clinically trained physicians. Because of the difficulty in being absolutely sure of the diagnosis, a doubtful category was established. When the examining physician made a diagnosis in this category, a second examiner's opinion was requested.

Physicians in clinical practice for the most part take care of patients who present themselves with relatively advanced disease. These individuals do not seek medical attention until the symptoms become sufficiently bothersome. For this reason most physicians are inclined to believe that the diagnosis of angina pectoris is relatively easy. By the time the patient seeks a medical opinion, the nature of the chest discomfort and the factors that relate to its appearance and disappearance can be well described. When the general public is evaluated, not those seeking medical care for chest discomfort, the problem is quite different. Large numbers of adults (up to 20 percent of the population) complain of some type of chest discomfort. In most, the pain is readily assessed as not that of angina pectoris. However, a considerable number of subjects have a degree of discomfort that requires a careful medical history before any conclusion can be reached.

Myocardial Infarction

The manifestation of coronary heart disease that has received most attention and is of most concern to the public is myocardial infarction. It is commonly referred to as a "heart attack," although that term includes also episodes involving similar symptoms without resultant infarction of the myocardium (then often labeled insufficiency).

A myocardial infarction results when prolonged ischemia of a segment of the myocardium leads to necrosis of that part of the muscle mass. Conceivably, recurrent ischemia might cause the destruction of occasional muscle cells and thus gradually lead to sufficient loss of functioning muscle fibriles that contractility is impaired, eventually leading to heart failure. However, the major manifestation of prolonged ischemia caused by severe narrowing or obstruction of the coronary artery is the death of a distinct mass of the myocardium and the accompanying symptoms and clinical signs of this event.

Considerable debate still exists about the exact train of pathological changes in the coronary circulation that lead to ischemia sufficiently severe and prolonged to cause myocardial necrosis. For many years it was believed that a thrombotic occlusion of a coronary artery or branch thereof was responsible. Myocardial infarction thus was commonly referred to as "coronary thrombosis" and the victim was said to have had a "coronary."

More recently it has become apparent that myocardial infarction can occur without thrombotic occlusion. Even when a thrombus is found at autopsy, the time the thrombus occurred is often questionable; many of the observed thromboses may have followed the infarction rather than causally preceding it. Of one fact we can be sure: myocardial infarction results from ischemia caused by atherosclerotic damage to the coronary artery. This damage may be solely in the form of atheromata that impinge on the lumen of the coronary arteries severely restricting blood flow. For the ischemia to produce clinical symptoms of angina pectoris, at least 70 percent narrowing of the arterial lumen is usually required. Even without significant narrowing of the coronary artery, atheromatous plaques on the walls may set the stage for thrombus formation; a true coronary artery thrombosis then occurs with sudden and essentially complete loss of blood supply to varying amounts of the myocardium. Myocardial infarction may, however, take place with only minimal narrowing of the coronary artery and without a visible thrombus at the time of autopsy.

Symptomatology of Myocardial Infarction

Myocardial infarction is accompanied by a wide range of clinical symptoms. In a small percentage, absolutely no symptoms can be recalled by those persons later discovered to have suffered a myocardial infarction by reason of characteristic diagnostic electrocardiographic findings at a routine examination. At the other extreme are persons who develop severe chest pain, shock, and a rapid demise because of massive myocardial necrosis.

The wide range of symptomatology of those patients *whose illness causes them to seek medical help* is well known to practicing physicians. They are, however, not familiar with those subjects who develop disease but do not seek medical attention for reasons that range from complete absence of any symptomatology ("silent" myocardial infarction) to classical manifestations of myocardial infarction in an extremely stoical person who accepts considerable discomfort without complaint. The symptoms may also be of such a bizarre or unusual type as to be interpreted to indicate some other disease that is not life threatening—pain felt mostly in the wrist and attributed by both patient and physician to joint or skeletal muscle disease. In the Framingham Study all patients found to have had a myocardial infarction but undiagnosed for whatever reason were categorized as "unrecognized" myocardial infarction.

One of the major contributions of epidemiologic studies is the opportunity to observe the complete course of the natural history of the disease. Such studies evaluate entire populations regardless of the presence or absence of symptomatology or the severity of it. An example of this can be seen in an analysis of the subjects developing myocardial infarction in the Framingham Study on the basis of recognition of the disease (Dawber and Stokes, 1959; Kannel et al., 1970; Margolis et al., 1973). In this group approximately 25 percent of patients developing myocardial infarction were unrecognized at the time the event occurred. Of these, half were considered to be completely asymptomatic. A later diagnosis of myocardial infarction was dependent on the development of diagnostic electrocardiographic changes not previously present. The percentage of patients with unrecognized myocardial infarction who were missed is undoubtedly minimal, since only a few subjects could have had this condition with return of the electrocardiographic changes to a nondiagnostic state before their biennial visit. The availability of the subjects' ECGs taken prior to the episode was of utmost importance in the determination of any interim myocardial infarction.

Most patients developing myocardial infarction survive long enough to describe their symptoms. The major one is the rather rapid onset of substernal or epigastric discomfort. In patients who have had angina pectoris the symptoms may seem very similar. Instead of disappearing, however, with rest or the administration of nitroglycerin, the symptoms persist and become more severe. The discomfort is often described as a crushing weight upon the chest. Pain may radiate into the neck, jaws, or down the arms. Persistence of the discomfort for more than a few minutes should alert both patient and physician that more than transient ischemia is occurring. In untreated survivors the discomfort may last several hours to one or two days, then gradually disappear. Patients in whom a diagnosis is made usually require pain relief for 24 to 72 hours. Since the chest discomfort is nonspecific and may be very similar to that observed in other serious disorders (such as dissection of the aorta, pulmonary embolism, and acute cholecystitis), it is necessary to make certain clinical tests to determine the underlying pathology. Fortunately the diagnostic procedures to confirm or rule out myocardial infarction are simple, safe, and highly accurate. These tests consist of electrocardiographic tracings taken serially during the first few days of the illness, certain enzyme tests that become positive during the period of acute necrosis, and other less specific findings such as elevated white blood count and increased sedimentation rate.

Of all the procedures the serial electrocardiogram is undoubtedly the most valuable. Without the development of the characteristic electrocardiographic changes of myocardial infarction it is difficult to be absolutely certain that such an event has occurred. For epidemiologic purposes, the investigator wishing to have unqualified objective evidence is justified in confining his definition of an incidence case of myocardial infarction to subjects who develop diagnostic electrocardiographic findings. In reaching the conclusion that a given electrocardiographic tracing is diagnostic of the development of a myocardial infarct, the investigator is greatly helped by having previous tracings taken on the same subject. Electrocardiographic tracings taken during periodic examinations serve as a baseline for concluding whether or not a new event has occurred and also determine whether what appear to be diagnostic Q waves have been present for many years or represent a new finding.

The sine qua non of myocardial infarction is the presence of Q waves not previously seen, and this has been the criterion of a diagnosis of myocardial infarction in the Framingham Study since its inception. One observation that may be of interest to those who have occasion to interpret electrocardiograms relates to the gradual appearance of Q waves over a number of years in asymptomatic and apparently disease-free subjects. A small number of participants in the Framingham Study have shown gradual increase in the width and depth of Q waves, particularly Q_{2-3} and Q_{AVF}, over many years until the electrocardiograms appear diagnostic of a previous myocardial infarction. The lack of other evidence that such an event had occurred and the very gradual appearance of these waves suggest that they are not indicative of a myocardial infarction. The cause of the Q-wave appearance is unknown. It is possible that repeated small areas of necrosis followed by fibrosis may eventually produce the same electrocardiographic patterns as a clinical myocardial infarction. In this study subjects developing the electrocardiographic changes described above have not been diagnosed as having developed myocardial infarction.

Enzyme Changes in Myocardial Infarction

With the necrosis of myocardial cells a number of enzymes normally present in these cells are released into the circulation. Measurement of these to aid in the diagnosis of myocardial infarction has now become a common laboratory service. At the time the Framingham Study was getting under way, this aid was not available. More recently, hospital records of patients with acute myocardial infarction contain data on a number of these enzymes that are used to establish the diagnosis.

Framingham Study subjects hospitalized for suspected myocardial infarction who presented evidence of sufficient rise in serum enzymes to warrant a diagnosis were classified as enzyme-positive myocardial infarction, whether or not diagnostic electrocardiographic findings were present. Diagnoses based only on clinical observations and positive enzyme studies with no electrocardiographic changes leave room for doubt about their validity. With typical patterns of enzyme rise and fall the physician may conclude that a myocardial infarction has occurred. However, other acute disorders may affect all the enzymes studied, so that the tests lack specificity and are primarily of value as confirmatory evidence.

Subjects diagnosed only on the basis of enzyme studies have been kept in a special category and comprise only about 10 percent of the total myocardial infarction population. I prefer, when possible, to confine analysis of myocardial infarction to those subjects showing positive electrocardiographic changes regardless of any enzyme findings.

Coronary Insufficiency

The term *coronary insufficiency* has been used with several different connotations. In one sense it merely implies an inadequate coronary arterial blood flow. Yet the term has also been loosely used as the basis for a number of nonspecific electrocardiographic changes not otherwise explained.

In the Framingham Study *coronary insufficiency* has been applied to a syndrome indistinguishable clinically from a myocardial infarction, except that no diagnostic electrocardiographic changes have developed—and no enzyme changes indicative of myocardial necrosis have been found. However, some positive objective evidence is required in the form of transient electrocardiographic changes. These changes are nonspecific but frequently include T-wave lowering, or inversion, and displacement of the S-T segment, often considered indicative of ischemia. Any changes found must disappear after a reasonable length of time. Many of the subjects diagnosed in this category have given histories of what may be called prolonged angina pectoris. The syndrome has also been designated *precoronary syndrome* or *intermediate syndrome*. The term *heart attack*, as commonly used, includes both myocardial infarction and coronary insufficiency. Sudden death and death caused by coronary heart disease (other than sudden) may also be referred to as heart attacks.

Sudden Death

The sudden collapse and death of an individual in apparently good health is a dramatic and shocking event that can have a number of causes. Most commonly, in Western countries, it results from sudden ischemia of the myocardium producing acute ventricular fibrillation or, less commonly, asystole. Pulmonary embolism and rupture or dissection of the aorta are two of the more common noncardiac causes.

Various studies of the underlying pathology of sudden death suggest that the present practice of considering all such deaths as caused by coronary artery disease unless proved otherwise is warranted. This is particularly true if the time interval required to define "sudden" death is brief. In the Framingham Study we decided to include only those subjects in the category of sudden death who had been observed to be in apparent good health but who *expired within one hour* of such observation. Any preexisting condition in which sudden death might be expected would not have been counted. Thus a patient with a known previous myocardial infarction who died suddenly would not be listed as a sudden death, since he already had a disease in which such a terminal event might be expected. A requirement of the definition of sudden death as used in this study was not only that it be sudden, but that it be unexpected from any known pathological condition already present.

The total number of persons dying suddenly will clearly be much higher than that based on the above definition. The use of one hour since apparent good health for a definition of "sudden" death is arbitrary. Other time limits, up to 24 hours, have been used (Gould, 1960). Unfortunately the longer the interval the greater the error in concluding that the underlying disorder is coronary artery disease.

Previous generations of physicians were taught to believe that the sudden collapse and death of an adult was frequently the result of a massive cerebral hemorrhage or infarction. Sudden death thus was frequently attributed to a cerebral vascular accident. Only in relatively recent times has there been recognition of the fact that extremely few such events resulted in death in less than 12 to 24 hours. Presumably if the 24-hour definition were to be used, a higher percentage of sudden deaths could reasonably be attributed to cerebral vascular accidents or other noncoronary artery diseases. In practice, it is often difficult to obtain precise information regarding the time sequence of death —particularly when the individual in question lived alone. The most frequent problem relates to the subject found dead who had not been seen alive for a number of hours. Very often, however, a careful description of the circumstances under which he was found will greatly improve our conclusions regarding the suddenness of death.

Although the presumption of coronary artery atherosclerosis of a significant degree is warranted when sudden death occurs, there have been a limited number of episodes of sudden death in which no findings of coronary artery pathology are reported. These occurrences are sufficiently infrequent that they do not invalidate the classification of sudden death as a manifestation of coronary heart disease.

Coronary Heart Disease Death Other Than Sudden

Death from coronary heart disease frequently occurs more than an hour following the onset of symptoms but before it has been possible to establish a definitive diagnosis. The symptomatology is strongly indicative of myocardial infarction or severe coronary insufficiency. Under such circumstances the assignment of the cause of death to coronary heart disease appears reasonable. Such deaths are frequently recorded as myocardial infarction on death certificates. We have chosen to place them in a special category of "coronary heart disease death—not sudden."

Atherosclerotic Cerebral Vascular Disease

The blood supply to the cerebrum involves not only the arterial tree within the skull but also the carotid, subclavian, and basilar arteries in the neck. These vessels should be considered as an important part of the cerebral arterial system. Emboli can originate also in the ascending aorta and in the heart—frequently from endocardial thrombi.

Study of the epidemiology of atherosclerotic cerebral vascular disease is complicated by the fact that although thrombotic disease is apparently the most common type of cerebral vascular accident, embolic obstruction is also frequent. Intracerebral hemorrhage and subarachnoid hemorrhage also occur with sufficient frequency that they must be considered in the differential diagnosis. All of these various pathological entities may produce clinical syndromes, which may be difficult to distinguish even after careful evaluation of all the facts (including autopsy findings).

Embolism to and rupture of the coronary arteries are extremely unusual, but because these pathological disorders frequently affect the cerebral vessels they pose a real problem in the differential diagnosis of cerebral vascular accidents. In some reports of the epidemiology of cerebral vascular disease no attempt has been made to separate the several entities. When the importance of certain precursors, such as elevated blood pressure, is considered, grouping all cerebral vascular accidents together may not invalidate the findings, for the correlation between elevated blood pressure and both thrombotic stroke and cerebral hemorrhage is very high. For most of the other factors, however, the inclusion of several unrelated pathological states in one clinical entity may invalidate any conclusions reached. For this reason we have endeavored in the Framingham Study to classify all cerebral vascular episodes under the following rubrics:

> Atherothrombotic brain infarction;
> Intracerebral hemorrhage;
> Subarachnoid hemorrhage;
> Cerebral embolism;
> Transient ischemic attacks.

Not until ten years after the initiation of this study was a decision made to include cerebral vascular disease as an endpoint for investigation. The incidence of cerebral vascular accidents in the young to middle-aged population is low relative to coronary heart disease, so that without the prospect of following a population well into older age epidemiologic studies of these disorders may be unrewarding.

Cerebral vascular disease involves a somewhat older population although, as will be discovered, the age differential is not so great as many physicians believe. The diagnosis that a cerebral vascular accident has occurred, especially if a significant neurological deficit has resulted, may not be hard to establish but determination of the underlying pathology, as indicated above, may be extremely difficult. The Framingham Study was fortunate to have the services of a neurologist interested in the epidemiologic aspect of cerebral vascular disease (Dr. Philip A. Wolf of the Boston University School of Medicine). He has reviewed the records of all cases suspected of having developed this disorder in any of its manifestations and, when possible, has made a clinical evaluation.

The difficulty in distinguishing between cerebral thrombosis and cerebral embolism is recognized. To a certain degree the distinction has been arbitrary, but it has been made according to a pattern that can be duplicated by other investigators.

Atherothrombotic Brain Infarction

This clinical entity is frequently referred to as cerebral thrombosis or thrombotic stroke. Although neuropathologists disagree on the underlying events, they generally agree that in most instances the development of brain infarction follows a course similar to that of myocardial infarction. Atherosclerotic plaques develop in the arteries leading to and within the brain, narrowing these vessels and setting up a nidus for thrombus formation. With sufficient narrowing of the carotid, basilar, and vertebral arteries or branches thereof, transient ischemic attacks may occur. This manifestation of cerebral vascular disease is comparable to angina pectoris. With the development of a thrombotic occlusion, permanent ischemia of a segment of the brain is produced and causes a *cerebral infarction*.

The clinical manifestations of cerebral infarction are dependent on the size of the infarct and its location in the brain. A minute infarction involving the brain stem might produce marked symptoms owing to dysfunction of the cranial nerves. A larger infarction of the brain, not involving the motor nerves, might occur without producing immediately recognizable effects.

In the Framingham Study the definition of brain infarction required the sudden appearance of a recognizable neurological deficit that lasted for at least 24 hours. It is important to realize that many patients who develop such manifestations are not sufficiently ill to require hospitalization. The number of persons hospitalized for this disorder might vary considerably depending on the customary medical practice. In Framingham most of those developing such symptoms were hospitalized for study. The inclusion of *all* subjects developing such findings, as compared to only those hospitalized or dying from them, might account for the somewhat higher incidence rates of this disorder in the Framingham Study than reported elsewhere.

INTRACEREBRAL HEMORRHAGE

A common cause of stroke is the rupture of an intracranial artery with hemorrhage into the brain substance. As with atherothrombotic brain infarction, there is the sudden development of a neurological deficit, usually of severe degree, often producing a rapidly developing comatose state. Distinction on clinical grounds between intracerebral hemorrhage and atherothrombotic brain infarction may be very difficult.

It was formerly taught that intracerebral hemorrhage was without exception a fatal event. It is now recognized that a small percentage of patients with this pathology may develop a hemorrhagic cyst, which destroys only a small volume of the brain tissue consistent with survival. Such subjects may be indistinguishable from those with brain infarction and may not develop bloody spinal fluid. In clinical practice in the past, the major factor in distinguishing cerebral hemorrhage from brain infarction was the finding of red blood cells in the spinal fluid, usually in grossly visible amounts. This has been the criterion used in the Framingham Study: the definition of intracerebral hemorrhage has been the sudden development of a neurological deficit in which blood has been found on spinal fluid examination. Clearly the distinction between intracerebral and subarachnoid hemorrhage may be difficult, for hemorrhagic spinal fluid is characteristic of both these entities. The similarity of clinical manifestations of intracerebral hemorrhage, subarachnoid hemorrhage, cerebral embolism, and brain infarction—in spite of completely different pathology of the cerebral arteries—is one confounding problem in the epidemiologic study of stroke. For this reason the study of "stroke" as an entity, although a useful exercise, cannot be as productive as the study of the different clinical pathological entities that constitute the all-inclusive group. As will be seen, it is reasonable to examine the relationship of such factors as elevated blood pressure using all stroke categories, since this factor so obviously relates to both thrombosis and hemorrhage.

Subarachnoid Hemorrhage

Hemorrhage caused by rupture of an aneurysm in the Circle of Willis discharges blood directly into the subarachnoid space. Damage to the brain results from compression and not from dissection and destruction as in intracerebral hemorrhage. Usually the symptoms are slower to develop and do not localize. Unsteadiness, lack of coordination, and slow response—often mistaken for acute alcoholism or other toxic disorders—may be the major manifestations. Gross blood in the spinal fluid is an early and rapid finding. Subjects with severe subarachnoid hemorrhage may be indistinguishable from those with intracerebral hemorrhage.

Cerebral Embolism

When emboli are carried into the cerebral circulation and block one or more of the cerebral vessels, an acute ischemia results that is indistinguishable from that produced by a thrombotic occlusion. The distinction between cerebral embolism and thrombosis, although important, is extremely difficult to make. The decision regarding which of these pathological entities is responsible for a neurological deficit is bound to be open to criticism.

In the Framingham Study all subjects developing strokes who for any reason had discharged emboli into the cerebral arterial circulation were considered to have had cerebral embolism. Thus persons developing strokes who were also diagnosed as having atrial fibrillation or who had had recent myocardial infarctions (within the previous six months) were classified as having cerebral embolism. Admittedly, not included were those individuals with atheromatous lesions of the ascending aorta, subclavian, and carotid arteries, portions of which could break free from the arterial wall and be carried farther into the cerebral circulation, eventually producing atheromatous embolic occlusion.

Until recent years this possibility had not received much attention, yet as pointed out above, emboli from atheromatous arterial lesions must certainly occur and very likely do so more frequently than has been believed. Some critics may object to the relatively low incidence of cerebral embolism in our series and believe that many of the subjects classified as atherothrombotic brain infarction had atheromatous emboli rather than thromboses. From the standpoint of studying atherosclerosis, this is not so serious a problem as the confusion between hemorrhage and thrombosis. There is no argument about the identity of the underlying atherosclerotic pathology, whether labeled thrombus or embolus.

Transient Ischemic Attacks

Very frequently the first manifestation of atherosclerotic cerebral vascular disease is the onset of transient ischemic attacks. A diagnosis of this disorder is often difficult because the physician seldom has an opportunity to actually observe the event. The episodes consist in fleeting periods of loss of consciousness or in inability to perform motor functions normally. Differentiation from fainting spells or epileptiform seizures may be extremely difficult.

Certain neurological deficits, such as transient monocular blindness representing ischemia caused by narrowing of the ophthalmic artery, are sufficiently characteristic as to be diagnostic; they are not readily confused with other nonvascular disorders. Transient ischemic attacks vary in frequency and quite often are followed by a thrombotic occlusion at differing time intervals. The diagnosis of cerebral disorders resulting from circulatory system disease is usually not difficult. The sine qua non is their sudden onset, their association with known cardiac disease, or the suspicion of cerebral arterial disease.

Peripheral Arterial Disease

The third major category of atherosclerotic disease involves the arteries of the lower extremity. Atherosclerotic changes in the aorta, the iliac, femoral, and popliteal arteries produce narrowing and occlusion with resultant ischemia of the feet and legs. This may cause gangrene (infarction), but much more frequently produces transient symptoms of ischemia. These symptoms are referred to as intermittent claudication and usually are felt in the calf muscles, less frequently in the thigh.

Intermittent claudication is described by the patient as a cramp, an ache, or tightness in the calf muscles. It is induced only by use of the leg muscles, generally by walking. After walking a variable distance, the patient notes onset of the discomfort. Stopping for only a few minutes relieves the symptom, which may recur upon resuming the muscular activity. The symptom is akin to and sometimes labeled angina of the legs. In eliciting this symptom, care must be taken not to confuse it with the leg aches noted *after* walking or bicycling long distances. The latter type of fatigue is not related to vascular disease, whereas typical intermittent claudication is diagnostic of occlusive disease of the lower extremities, almost always the result of atherosclerotic narrowing and frequently thrombosis of the leg arteries. Although other relatively rare disorders may produce this symptom, in the adult population intermittent claudication is essentially synonymous with peripheral arteriosclerosis. Attempts have been made to provide more objective methods of diagnosing peripheral arterial disease. Textbooks on the subject always refer to palpation of the peripheral vessels and suggest that diminished or absent pulsation in the dorsalis pedis or posterior tibial arteries is of great importance in the diagnosis. However, the variability of pulsations in these vessels in healthy individuals is so great that this criterion is virtually useless. The exception would be the *disappearance* of pulsations in a patient in whom they had previously been present.

Attempts have been made to record pulsations mechanically or electronically. In the Framingham Study a pulse wave recorder was used. This device compared the pulsations at several points on both legs, on the assumption that they would rarely show the same degree of occlusive disease. Data from this procedure confirmed symptoms of claudication but did not furnish sufficient additional information to warrant the effort.

For diagnostic purposes in the Framingham Study the identification of symptoms of intermittent claudication was the determinant of peripheral arterial disease and therefore the only category established.

Congestive Heart Failure

Diagnoses of congestive heart failure were based on findings from the biennial examination and/or from hospital records. In order that the diagnosis be standardized, lists of major and minor criteria were developed. A diagnosis of definite congestive heart failure required the presence of two major or one major and two minor criteria (McKee et al., 1971). For practical purposes almost all the subjects had evidence of pulmonary congestion and heart enlargement by x-ray, and electrocardiographic evidence of left ventricular hypertrophy. For classification purposes probable and questionable categories were also established.

Hypotheses for Study

4

ONCE THE CRITERIA for diagnosis of the disorders to be studied have been established, the next task of the epidemiologic investigator is to determine what characteristics of host and environment are worth examining in relation to disease development. It is unlikely that a study would be contemplated at all without the existence of some plausible hypotheses linking certain host or environmental characteristics to disease. But hypotheses are frequently developed without careful consideration of the feasibility of putting them to a test. When the time for proving them arrives, the investigator may have difficulty finding a practicable means of conducting the necessary research. One of the major roles of an investigator is the translation of a general hypothesis into specific terms that will permit conduct of an investigation to test it.

In the initial planning of our study a series of hypotheses was developed. The task of the Framingham investigators, where possible, was to attempt to prove these hypotheses. If direct testing were not feasible, other hypotheses might be generated that would shed light on the subject without necessarily answering the original question proposed. Our major hypotheses are presented in this section, along with some of the detailed considerations to be discussed in subsequent chapters.

The establishment of the hypotheses and their expression in

such a way that an investigation can be conducted to test their validity is of utmost importance. Two aspects of this problem are worthy of consideration: (1) the hypotheses should be rational and based on such scientific knowledge of the subject as is available at the time; and (2) a hypothesis that relates a characteristic of host or environment to the development of a disease entity must be formulated with concern both for the quantitative and qualitative measurement of the disease and the suspected risk factor; in other words, both the occurrence of disease and the presence of the risk factors must be measurable. That a hypothesis currently appears reasonable does not preclude the possibility that later knowledge of the subject may make it seem less so, or vice versa. However, the more solidly a hypothesis is based on existing fact or reasonable belief, the more likely it will be supported by tests of its validity.

In the development of the Framingham Study a great deal of thought went into the selection of hypotheses for investigation. These were determined by the staff, with substantial input from an advisory committee composed of specialists representing several branches of medical science. This committee had a high proportion of practicing cardiologists with long experience in atherosclerotic disease, who from time to time had observed apparent relationships between certain host and environmental characteristics and the presence of cardiovascular disease.

Physicians observe and record a number of characteristics of persons with already overt disease. Whether the characteristics are specifically associated with the disease is often a matter of impression, since comparative groups of nondiseased individuals are not usually available for examination. Furthermore, an association with overt disease does not necessarily indicate correlation with its initial development. In spite of these reservations the impressions of physicians, who are careful observers, about factors that relate to disease must be taken seriously.

Specific Hypotheses Formulated for Testing

(1) Coronary heart disease increases with age (as do other manifestations of atherosclerotic disease). It occurs earlier and more frequently in the male sex.

Observation of practicing physicians and such vital statistics as were available suggested strongly that coronary heart disease was largely a male disease and that it increased steadily with age. It was quite rare under age 30. Although there was little reason to believe that the observations already made would be contradicted by the Framingham findings, quantitation was considered desirable. The suggestion that the study be confined to men because of the reported low prevalence and incidence in women was rejected; we believed that this sex difference might provide a valuable clue to other factors that might prove to be causally related.

(2) Persons with hypertension develop coronary heart disease at a greater rate than those who are normotensive.

A sizable body of knowledge previously collected by insurance companies indicated a higher mortality rate in persons with elevated blood pressure (Proc. Assoc. Life Ins. Med. Dirs. America, 1942). The data applied primarily to subjects with excessively high blood pressure. The general impression was that persons developing a disease—"hypertension"—were destined to get into cardiovascular difficulty, but that there were many people with "benign" hypertension in whom blood-pressure elevation was either harmless or not associated with a significantly excessive risk. The concept was that blood pressure per se did not present a hazard, regardless of the level, but that instead the untoward effects were caused by an underlying "disease," of which elevated blood pressure was one prominent manifestation.

(3) Elevated blood cholesterol level is associated with an increased risk of coronary heart disease.

Evidence at the time of planning the Framingham Study supported the belief that persons with serious lipid disorders, particularly familial hypercholesterolemia, were at high risk of atherosclerotic disease (Adlersberg, Parets, and Boas, 1949). Such individuals had blood cholesterol levels that were extremely high (600 mg % or more). The same consideration was accorded hypercholesterolemia as hypertension—that there might well be "benign" hypercholesterolemia and that in the absence of a hypercholesterolemic "disease" (familial xanthomatosis) the finding of elevated serum cholesterol might have no importance. It was decided that this hypothesis required careful investigation.

At the initiation of the study the practicability of exploring factors relating to cholesterol levels was not apparent. Several years later, when the study was firmly established, the feasibility of investigating the major environmental factor proposed—dietary intake—was considered. As a result, a program was undertaken to test the hypothesis that fat and cholesterol in the diet were related to serum cholesterol level.

(4) Tobacco smoking is associated with an increased occurrence of coronary heart disease.

At the time the Framingham Study was organized, there was no convincing evidence of the hazard of tobacco smoking insofar as coronary heart disease was concerned. On theoretical grounds, the known acute effects of nicotine in temporarily elevating blood pressure, pulse rate, and cardiac output, and the effects of smoking in increasing myocardial irritability, suggested a possibility that chronic damage might also be produced (English, Willius, and Berkson, 1940; Roth and Shick, 1958). There was certainly no convincing evidence of an increased rate or atherosclerosis in tobacco users.

There can be no doubt that physicians and nonmedical people alike looked with disfavor on the use of tobacco long before the early evidence of a link with lung cancer incidence. Some of this attitude was related to a common belief that the use of stimulants (nicotine) was inherently immoral. By 1950 evidence had already been accumulated that indicated a higher incidence rate of lung cancer in cigarette smokers (Doll and Hill, 1950). This finding, together with the known acute effects of nicotine on the cardiovascular system, made more plausible the assumption that smoking might be related to other diseases and encouraged further investigation of the hypothesis.

(5) Habitual use of alcohol is associated with increased incidence of coronary heart disease.

Data already were available suggesting a higher mortality rate from a number of causes in alcoholics (Schmidt and DeLint, 1972). In addition, a myopathy of undetermined origin was occasionally observed in habitual, excessive alcohol users (McKinney, 1974). Since alcohol is a toxic agent, there was good reason to believe that it might have an adverse effect on the heart; by damaging the arterial intima it could conceivably relate to the development or progression of atherosclerotic plaque (Grollman, 1930). The prevailing belief was that alcoholic intake contributes only minimally to the atherosclerotic process.

(6) Increased physical activity is associated with a decrease in the development of coronary heart disease.

Although this hypothesis was not included in the original list, it was added shortly after initiation of the study. There were conflicting opinions regarding the benefit of hard physical work or high-energy-output exercise on the cardiovascular system. One of the members of the advisory committee was of the opinion that those doing hard physical work or habitually engaged in vigorous physical exercise would have higher rates of coronary heart disease (Levine and Brown, 1929). This was because of the marked effect of increased physical activity on blood-pressure elevation. Such elevation (at least systolic), observed in athletes while performing vigorous exercise, resembled that measured in persons with known hypertension. This opinion was countered by those who believed that there was metabolic advantage to be derived from increasing the total metabolism by raising the energy output. This benefit might be akin to that of hyperthyroidism in lowering blood cholesterol. In view of the difference of opinion regarding the possible hazard or benefit of increased physical activity, a decision was made to attempt to determine the effect of this variable on the development of coronary heart disease, although the difficulty of making the necessary measurements was recognized.

(7) An increase in thyroid function is associated with a decrease in the development of coronary heart disease.

There was evidence that subjects with clinically recognizable hypothyroidism had higher levels of serum cholesterol, and there was also a belief, admittedly unsubstantiated, that persons with hypothyroidism developed angina pectoris and myocardial infarction more frequently. On the other side was the knowledge that a decrease in metabolic rate was often accompanied by the disappearance of angina pectoris in patients so afflicted. Both surgical thyroidectomy and radiation of the thyroid were employed for the disorder—with some success, but not without criticism.

    (8) A high blood hemoglobin or hematocrit level is associated with an increased rate of development of coronary heart disease.

There was some evidence suggesting that persons with polycythemia were at increased risk of stroke, and less convincing evidence that the same was true for myocardial infarction. However, the increased viscosity and probable hypercoagulability observed in polycythemia could reasonably be connected to higher thrombotic incidence and could possibly contribute to the development of atherosclerotic plaques.

    (9) An increase in body weight predisposes to coronary heart disease.

There was already substantial evidence that overweight individuals had a higher death rate and that a considerable number of the excess deaths were attributable to coronary heart disease and other atherosclerotic disorders (Levy et al., 1946). Insurance-company data were the primary source of knowledge concerning the hazards of excess weight.

    (10) There is an increased rate of development of coronary heart disease in patients with diabetes mellitus.

The high rate of cardiovascular complications in juvenile diabetes was well recognized. The evidence that mature-onset diabetes was associated with higher incidence of these complications was suggestive, but not proven (Root et al., 1939).

    (11) There is a higher incidence of coronary heart disease in patients with gout.

There was a clinical belief that these two disorders were associated because of the underlying metabolic disorder of uric acid.

A number of minor hypotheses was also proposed, and from time to time additional hypotheses were considered. Genetic relationships were believed to be of importance, but their inclusion in the study was not considered feasible.

Incidence of Coronary Heart Disease, Stroke, and Peripheral Arterial Disease

5

THE POPULATION FOR STUDY was selected with the thought that data on prevalence and incidence of the various clinical entities would be applicable to much larger populations, including that of the United States as a whole. Yet because of incomplete participation of the selected sample, the Framingham investigators were hesitant afterward to publish reports on their findings of the prevalence of cardiovascular disorders. There was no doubt that the presence of overt disease was an important factor in discouraging participation in the study. Those persons who had previously developed cardiovascular disease and who were already under medical care had little reason to enroll in a research project that was not concerned with therapeutic intervention. Similarly, those with other serious diseases saw no benefit to themselves accruing from participation in a study of cardiovascular disease which they probably would not live long enough to develop. Any report of the prevalence of the atherosclerotic diseases undoubtedly would have seriously underestimated the true figures. Unless a comprehensive house-to-house survey of the nonparticipants had been conducted, reliable data on prevalence could not have been obtained. However, as part of the public relations approach in the community, it had been agreed that no personal visits to households would be conducted. Because of the possible lack of reliability of the prevalence data and the primary concern with incidence of disease, we decided to await the occurrence of new disease before trying to estimate the magnitude of the coronary heart disease problem.

The failure of total participation may also affect the incidence figures. Since subjects who elect to participate in medical research projects are ipso facto more interested in health matters than those who refuse, these individuals may not be completely representative of the total population. The better health experience usually observed in such study groups suggests that estimates of incidence data obtained from them may be lower than if there had been total participation.

In spite of these uncertainties, there appears to be good reason to accept the Framingham findings as a reliable estimate of the actual incidence of the various disorders, with some obvious exceptions: there were too few black residents of Framingham to provide sufficient incidence data; the makeup of the white population was not completely representative of the U.S. white population: and there were more participants of Italian extraction than would be found in most communities in this country. However, unless national origin plays an important role (which apparently it does not), the data reported may be considered reasonably representative of the North American white population.

The incidence of atherosclerotic disease was known to be age related, increasing with age in each sex (Winter et al., 1958). The absolute incidence rises with the length of the observation period. As subjects pass through a given age span, they contribute to the rate of development of disease in that interval. A new population at risk is constantly being generated from the younger cohort from which fresh cases of disease will occur. The average annual rate will not change significantly regardless of the observation period, once sufficient data are available for adequate analysis.

Incidence may be described as the amount of disease that develops out of a given population at risk followed for a specified time. Incidence may also be calculated for short age ranges and include all members of the population passing through the given age brackets. If the observation period is a long one, as in the Framingham Study, an average annual incidence rate for older age groups will make use of larger numbers of the population, as the younger subjects move into the older ages.

The tables on incidence of atherosclerotic disease are based on the first 24 years of our study and indicate the actual (crude) rates measured during this period. The total incidence will increase still further until all subjects have developed disease or have died. The age-specific rates will not be perceptibly affected by longer observation unless more numbers are needed to determine validity.

In addition, the crude rates have been corrected to take into account those members of the population who are no longer at risk by reason of having developed the disorder in question or having been lost to observation by death. The crude rate can be used as an estimate of developing disease, if we assume the usual rates of death from other causes. The corrected rate provides an estimate of the "true" risk if no other disorders have intervened.

Analysis of data in epidemiologic studies usually begins with observations on the relation of the age and sex of the subjects at risk to disease development. The aging process is still not well understood. Very clearly, cells—even in tissue cultures—change with age and with repeated reproduction. These alterations may be caused solely by the aging process. However, it is also possible that in many instances what has been considered purely a function of this aging process may in fact be the result of prolonged exposure to noxious influences. Increasing age might thus reflect prolonged exposure to a number of factors that over a brief period have had little impact. Many years of exposure could produce irreparable damage. The concept of a time-dose relationship is readily understandable and may be the explanation for many of the bodily changes now attributed to aging. If we acknowledge that tissues do change with age, it is understandable that many factors may either accelerate or retard the aging process in general and have specific effects on certain of the pathological processes considered part of aging.

Atherosclerosis has been accepted as one of the pathological changes related to age (White, Edwards, and Day, 1950). Only a few individuals who survive to very old age are relatively free of this disorder, and in general both the area of the arterial walls involved and the state of the atheromatous plaque are age related.

Physicians in clinical practice have long recognized that heart attacks and sudden death have been more frequent and have occurred earlier in life in men than in women (Master, Dack, and Jaffe, 1939). The magnitude of the difference had not been fully documented, and the reasons for the sex difference were speculative. At the start of the Framingham Study it was widely believed that the atherosclerotic process progressed at a slower rate in women than men and that the clinical manifestations of the disorder were encountered much less frequently in women. The observation of a marked sex difference in incidence of coronary heart disease led many investigators to focus attention almost entirely on the male sex.

Because of the apparent difference in the incidence rates in men and women, we felt that an epidemiologic study involving both sexes might shed light on the reasons for this difference. Accordingly, provisions were made to include both men and women by enrolling family units in the population at risk.

Incidence of Clinical Manifestations of Atherosclerosis by Age and Sex

TOTAL CORONARY HEART DISEASE

Both age and sex were important factors in the 24-year incidence of coronary heart disease (Fig. 5-1).* In men the incidence rates rose steadily with age by five-year brackets. A steeper rise was seen with the corrected figures, since by this method the estimated incidence in the higher age brackets more correctly reflected the "true" incidence rate. In the youngest cohort the crude and corrected rates were very similar. As might be expected, the average age at which disease occurred in the several age cohorts rose because of the higher average age of the population at risk.

Sex differences in incidence were marked. In the youngest decade the rate in men was three times that in women. The sex

---

*Unless otherwise specified, all the figures in this chapter and later ones are based on data collected over 24 years in the Framingham Study.

difference became smaller with increasing age, dropping to a ratio of 2.3 in the middle decade and to 1.7 in the 50-59 decade. For all ages (30-59) there was approximately twice the incidence of coronary heart disease in the men as in the women. Not only were the incidence rates higher at all ages for men, but the average age at which disease developed was approximately two years earlier. This age difference further emphasized the more frequent occurrence of the disease in males.

Myocardial Infarction

Myocardial infarction was the predominant clinical manifestation of coronary heart disease. Since this clinical entity is the one determined most objectively, the incidence data undoubtedly have the greatest validity. Within this category the validity can be still further refined by insistence on electrocardiographic changes diagnostic of the disorder. When we used this criterion, approximately one-fifth of all those with this diagnosis were removed (in other words, 80 percent of all myocardial infarction cases had unequivocal diagnostic electrocardiographic evidence). The percentage held in both sexes and at all ages.

The incidence rates of myocardial infarction by age groups over the 24-year period followed a pattern similar to that of total coronary heart disease (Figs. 5-2 and 5-3). The incidence rates rose steadily with age in both sexes. In the age groups studied there was no suggestion of peaking in any age span. The differences in the incidence rates in men and women at any age were much more striking than for total coronary heart disease. The increase in incidence with age was also considerably steeper in women than in men. As noted for all coronary heart disease, not only was myocardial infarction much more frequent in men, but the average age at which it developed was approximately two years earlier.

Sudden Death

The incidence of sudden death by age was proportionate to that observed in total coronary heart disease (Fig. 5-4). The incidence in the two sexes showed an even greater disparity than was evident in myocardial infarction. In men in the younger age groups the incidence rates of sudden death were approximately six times higher than in women. For the entire population the rate in men was about four times that observed in women. Sudden death on the average occurred approximately four years earlier in men than in women. When both the incidence rate and the age of occurrence were considered together, sudden death became an even greater hazard for men.

Angina Pectoris

The difference in incidence rates for angina pectoris between men and women, although less than observed in myocardial infarction or sudden death, was still substantial (Fig. 5-5). In the younger-age subjects observed for 24 years, there was about twice as much angina pectoris in the men as in the women. In the older subjects the ratio dropped to about one and one-half to one. As observed for other manifestations of coronary heart disease, the men developing angina pectoris were younger than the women in all age categories.

Other Manifestations of Coronary Heart Disease

The incidence rates for the other two manifestations of coronary heart disease—coronary insufficiency and death other than sudden—are presented in Figs. 5-6 and 5-7. The patterns are similar to total coronary heart disease, and the average age of onset was again earlier in men than in women.

Summary

In total coronary heart disease and in the several clinical entities that comprise this disorder, there is a clear-cut relation of incidence to age and a marked difference in incidence rates between the sexes. The average age of onset was significantly earlier in men. Coronary heart disease is predominantly a male disease: the difference in incidence was most pronounced in the younger ages, where the strong relationships of maleness to myocardial infarction and sudden death are noteworthy.

(*continued on page 68*)

INCIDENCE OF CORONARY HEART DISEASE

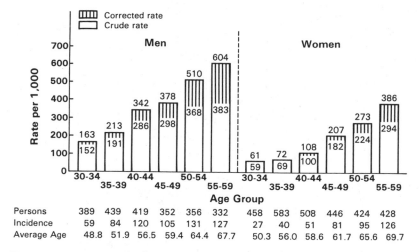

Fig. 5-1 *24-year incidence of coronary heart disease in men and women age 30-59 at entry.*

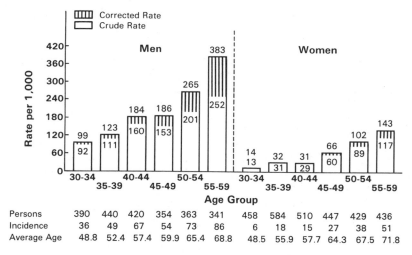

Fig. 5-2 *24-year incidence of myocardial infarction in men and women age 30-59 at entry.*

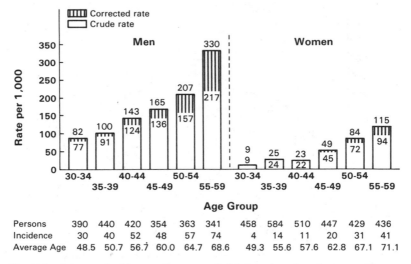

Persons	390	440	420	354	363	341	458	584	510	447	429	436
Incidence	30	40	52	48	57	74	4	14	11	20	31	41
Average Age	48.5	50.7	56.7	60.0	64.7	68.6	49.3	55.6	57.6	62.8	67.1	71.1

Fig. 5-3 *24-year incidence of myocardial infarction, by electrocardiogram, in men and women age 30-59 at entry.*

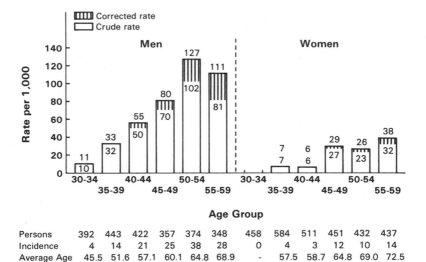

Persons	392	443	422	357	374	348	458	584	511	451	432	437
Incidence	4	14	21	25	38	28	0	4	3	12	10	14
Average Age	45.5	51.6	57.1	60.1	64.8	68.9	-	57.5	58.7	64.8	69.0	72.5

Fig. 5-4 *24-year incidence of sudden death in men and women age 30-59 at entry.*

INCIDENCE OF CORONARY HEART DISEASE

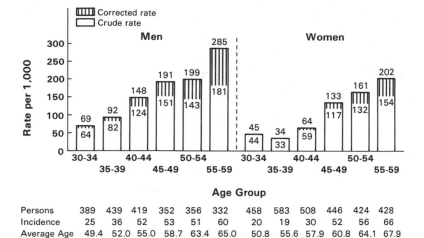

Persons	389	439	419	352	356	332	458	583	508	446	424	428
Incidence	25	36	52	53	51	60	20	19	30	52	56	66
Average Age	49.4	52.0	55.0	58.7	63.4	65.0	50.8	55.6	57.9	60.8	64.1	67.9

Fig. 5-5 *24-year incidence of angina pectoris in men and women age 30-59 at entry.*

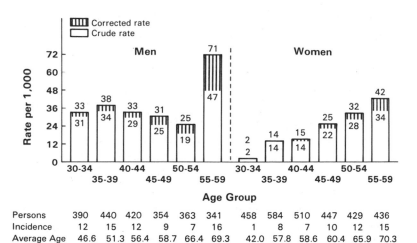

Persons	390	440	420	354	363	341	458	584	510	447	429	436
Incidence	12	15	12	9	7	16	1	8	7	10	12	15
Average Age	46.6	51.3	56.4	58.7	66.4	69.3	42.0	57.8	58.6	60.4	65.9	70.3

Fig. 5-6 *24-year incidence of coronary insufficiency in men and women age 30-59 at entry.*

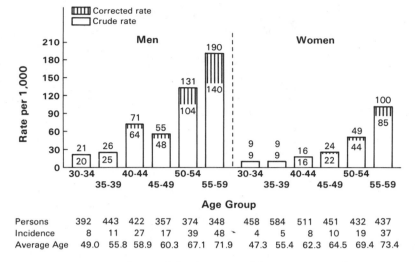

Fig. 5-7 *24-year incidence of death—not sudden—in men and women age 30-59 at entry.*

Cerebral Vascular Accidents (Stroke)

The several clinical entities grouped together under stroke or cerebral vascular accidents, with the problems in clinical differentiation, have been described in Chapter 3. Because of these difficulties, many investigators have preferred to use the all-inclusive category of stroke rather than the individual entities in studying the epidemiology of cerebral vascular disease. Stroke has long been recognized as a disease of older age in comparison with coronary heart disease, but age difference between the two disorders is often estimated to be greater than is warranted by actual observations (Fig. 5-8). Comparisons of the age of onset of stroke versus coronary heart disease showed that although the age was higher for stroke, in both sexes the difference was slight, amounting to only about two years. Comparison of the gradient of incidence with age shows a much steeper rise in all types of stroke. There was seven to ten times the stroke incidence in the oldest cohort followed for 24 years compared to the youngest. In contrast to the findings of a strong male predominance in coronary heart disease, the incidence of stroke in the two sexes was remarkably similar.

Atherothrombotic Brain Infarction

Atherothrombotic brain infarction constituted the largest category of cerebral vascular accidents. As discussed in Chapter 3, distinction between atherothrombotic brain infarction and cerebral embolism on clinical grounds may be impossible. In the Framingham classification cerebral embolism was diagnosed only when there was reason to suspect an embolic focus. As will be seen later, comparison of the relation of certain risk factors to both embolic disorders and thrombotic strokes suggested that the classification used was justified. When the analysis was confined to atherothrombotic brain infarction, the pattern was similar to that seen for all cerebral vascular accidents (Fig. 5-9). This was to be expected in view of the large percentage of the stroke category made up of patients with brain infarctions.

Whereas the overall rate was not significantly different in the two sexes, there was a slightly higher incidence of atherothrombotic brain infarction in younger men. The mean age at which such infarction occurred in men was very similar to that in women. The age difference between atherothrombotic brain infarction and myocardial infarction was about two years, much less than is generally believed. The marked difference in incidence of myocardial infarction in the two sexes was absent in atherothrombotic brain infarction, for reasons that are not apparent. The usual explanation of an older age of onset of atherothrombotic brain infarction compared to myocardial infarction was not applicable to the Framingham data.

Peripheral Arterial Disease

Intermittent Claudication

The only clinical manifestation of peripheral arterial disease used for the measurement of incidence was intermittent claudication. The relative incidence rates by age and sex followed a pattern similar to that of coronary heart disease (Fig. 5-10). The rates in the oldest decade were about four times those in the youngest, and the incidence in men was approximately twice that in women in each age group studied. Once again, the age of onset in men was about two years earlier than in women.

Interrelationships of the Atherosclerotic Diseases

In the presence of atherosclerotic disease in the arterial system of one part of the body, a greater degree of the same disease elsewhere in the vascular bed might be expected. The extent to which this occurs can be measured by observing the incidence of other manifestations of the disease developing in subjects in whom one clinical syndrome is already overt. Angina pectoris has been considered an earlier and possibly more benign manifestation of atherosclerotic coronary heart disease. For all forms of coronary heart disease other than angina pectoris, the average annual incidence rates were approximately two and one-half times higher in persons previously presenting symptoms of angina pectoris than in those free of this disorder (Fig. 5-11). In younger subjects this ratio was much higher (five to one).

The measurement of myocardial infarction occurring in subjects already presenting evidence of angina pectoris may be considered a reasonable estimate of the degree to which both are manifestations of the underlying coronary artery atherosclerosis. The average annual incidence rates of myocardial infarction in subjects with angina pectoris may be compared to the rates in those without this symptom (Fig. 5-12). For all ages the rate in those with angina was six times that of the nonanginal subjects. The difference in rates was greatest in the youngest persons and was similar in men and women. As a risk factor for the development of myocardial infarction, angina pectoris was the most potent.

The sudden-death rate in subjects with angina pectoris likewise was much higher (Fig. 5-13). The excess rates in the anginal subjects were even greater than for the other manifestations. This is understandable if our assumption is correct that both of these conditions are more truly reflections of transient ischemia resulting from coronary artery atherosclerosis than are some of the other manifestations.

Since both angina pectoris and intermittent claudication are strictly manifestations of transient ischemia, a positive association was expected and in fact was found (Fig. 5-14). The rate was approximately seven times greater in subjects with angina pectoris than in those with no anginal symptoms. Physicians may be inclined more readily to accept symptoms suggestive of intermittent claudication as indicative of this disorder in patients with known vascular disease. Cognizant of this bias, the examiners in Framingham were more careful in assigning a diagnosis of a second vascular manifestation. The figures presented, therefore, should not overstate the relationship of these two manifestations of ischemia.

Atherothrombotic brain infarction and myocardial infarction are comparable disorders in their respective organs. Myocardial infarction may through embolism be causally related to stroke. However, the occurrence of myocardial infarction in patients who have suffered a brain infarction suggests similarity of the underlying pathogenetic mechanism. In order to test this hypothesis, the entire category of stroke was needed to obtain enough cases for analysis. When the development of myocardial infarction was examined in those subjects who had suffered a stroke, the risk of developing a myocardial infarction was four times greater than in those in whom no cerebral vascular accident had occurred (Fig. 5-15).

From the above data we must conclude that in fact there is a strong association among the several categories of atherosclerotic disease. They are all markedly age related. The presence of one manifestation of atherosclerotic disease greatly increases the probability of developing another. And, as we shall see later, the risk factors contributing to one frequently also relate to another.

(Figures 5-8 to 5-15 follow)

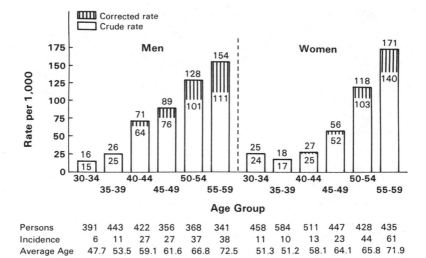

Persons	391	443	422	356	368	341	458	584	511	447	428	435
Incidence	6	11	27	27	37	38	11	10	13	23	44	61
Average Age	47.7	53.5	59.1	61.6	66.8	72.5	51.3	51.2	58.1	64.1	65.8	71.9

Fig. 5-8 *24-year incidence of cerebral vascular accident in men and women age 30-59 at entry.*

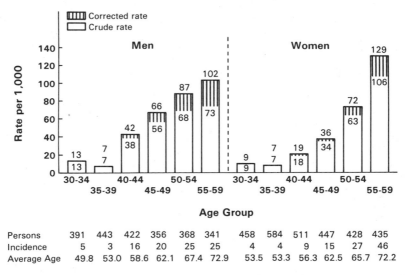

Persons	391	443	422	356	368	341	458	584	511	447	428	435
Incidence	5	3	16	20	25	25	4	4	9	15	27	46
Average Age	49.8	53.0	58.6	62.1	67.4	72.9	53.5	53.3	56.3	62.5	65.7	72.2

Fig. 5-9 *24-year incidence of atherothrombotic brain infarction in men and women age 30-59 at entry.*

INCIDENCE OF CORONARY HEART DISEASE

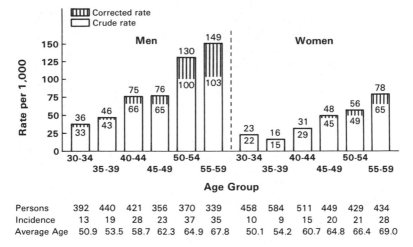

Persons	392	440	421	356	370	339	458	584	511	449	429	434
Incidence	13	19	28	23	37	35	10	9	15	20	21	28
Average Age	50.9	53.5	58.7	62.3	64.9	67.8	50.1	54.2	60.7	64.8	66.4	69.0

Fig. 5-10 *24-year incidence of intermittent claudication in men and women age 30-59 at entry.*

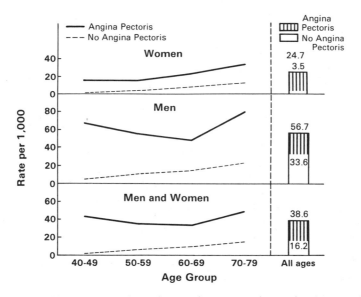

Fig. 5-11 *Average annual incidence of coronary heart disease in subjects with angina pectoris.*

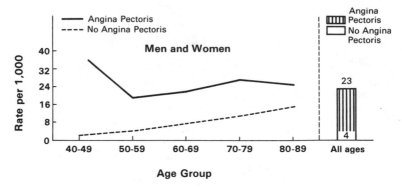

Fig. 5-12 *Average annual incidence of myocardial infarction in subjects with angina pectoris.*

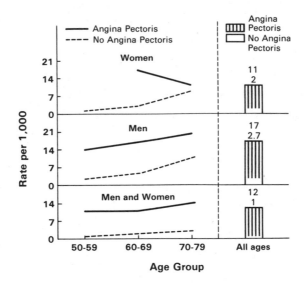

Fig. 5-13 *Average annual incidence of sudden death in subjects with angina pectoris.*

INCIDENCE OF CORONARY HEART DISEASE

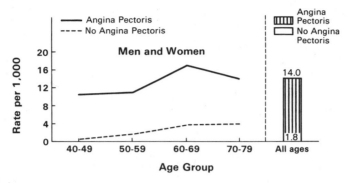

Fig. 5-14 *Average annual incidence of intermittent claudication in subjects with angina pectoris.*

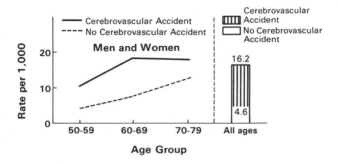

Fig. 5-15 *Average annual incidence of myocardial infarction in subjects with cerebral vascular accidents.*

Observations on
Blood-Pressure Measurement

6

ONE OF THE OBJECTIVES of the Framingham Study was to determine the epidemiology of hypertension; another was to study the effect that various blood-pressure levels might have on accelerating the atherosclerotic process. Elevation of blood pressure is a risk factor for atherosclerotic disease; it may also be considered a "disease" per se, since it may have severe cardiovascular complications unrelated to the atherosclerotic process—cerebral hemorrhage and congestive heart failure.

This chapter describes the course of blood-pressure changes in the Framingham Study population over the period of 24 years and indicates what factors, if any, played a role in elevating the pressure of some of the subjects. The original plan anticipated exclusion from further follow-up of all persons who on initial examination had evidence of existing coronary heart disease *or* hypertension (defined as a casual blood-pressure level of 160/95 mm Hg or higher). However, the opinion of the advisory committee was that by excluding subjects with already existing hypertension, we would lose an opportunity to determine the effect of blood-pressure elevation on subsequent cardiovascular disease. This decision was certainly wise in view of later findings of the importance of elevated blood-pressure level as a cardiovascular disease risk factor, and the nondevelopment of

OBSERVATIONS ON BLOOD-PRESSURE MEASUREMENT

many new cases of hypertension from those subjects whose blood pressure was initially low.

In approaching the subject of blood pressure and its effect on coronary heart disease and other atherosclerotic disorders, it is desirable to consider some of the problems of measurement, the distribution of blood-pressure levels in the study population, the correlation with age and sex, and other factors that may affect blood-pressure level (as opposed to the effect this level has on the development of atherosclerotic disease).

Definition of Hypertension

The term *hypertension* is an unfortunate one that should never have been introduced into medical terminology. It implies that anyone whose blood-pressure level has been recorded above an arbitrary value has a disease; that the population can be divided into those who have a disease, "hypertension," and those who do not. From the point of view of practicing physicians who must determine whether to treat or not, there needs to be a method of classifying patients to make possible this decision. Physicians have been trained to make basic decisions relating to the presence or absence of disease. Their entire program of history taking, physical examination, and laboratory studies is aimed at determining whether a disease can be found or whether the subject is "normal," which in medical usage means free of disease as determined by arbitrary definitions.

Since the blood pressure, as measured in the general population, may not be readily classified as either high or normal but follows a normal distribution curve, slightly skewed to the right, any designation of "normal," "high," or "borderline" is arbitrary. Considerable variability is included within each category. Thus the systolic blood pressure varied from 75 to 29 mm Hg when the Framingham Study population was first examined in 1950 to 1952. Within the arbitrarily designated "normotensive" subjects there was still a wide range of blood-pressure measurements, and within the "hypertensive" category an even wider range. Whenever an attempt is made to convert quantitative data to qualitative categories (to change continuous variables into discrete variables) a problem may arise. This is particularly true of the classification of blood-pressure measurement, because it causes both physician and patient to concentrate on whether or not a disease is present, rather than on maintaining as low a blood pressure as possible regardless of what the particular level may be. This problem has not been satisfactorily solved, even when dealing with diabetes mellitus, which is more clearly established as a disease although without a universally accepted definition. Whether blood-sugar measurements alone are sufficient criteria is debatable.

The measurement of blood pressure is further complicated by the variability of values within the same subject upon repeated examinations. This variability results from many factors. In some persons, particularly those with quite low pressures, there may be little variability throughout a 24-hour period or even at more prolonged intervals; in persons with higher pressures, the variability may be considerable.

Statisticians are often inclined to perceive the differences in recorded blood-pressure levels as *errors of measurement*, as if there were a fixed blood-pressure measurement assignable to each subject just as height or weight. The assigned value would not vary except within a small range, reflecting differences of measurement rather than differences of actual value. In view of the real variability of blood pressure in the same individual over short periods of time, it is necessary to describe carefully the circumstances under which the blood-pressure measurement was made. Successive determinations, for example, should be obtained under circumstances as nearly as identical as possible to those of the original determination with which they are to be compared. This becomes particularly important when therapeutic efforts are to be introduced to lower the pressure, and evaluation of the usefulness of the therapy is contemplated.

One of the major factors that temporarily elevates blood pressure is the anxiety of the patient about having the pressure measured. Every physician is aware that the pressure reading becomes lower and lower with successive determinations during a single examination period. Should he accept the first pressure recorded or the last as the "true" pressure? One customary procedure is to obtain a series of blood-pressure measurements and to record only the lowest. Many physicians do this when reporting blood-pressure measurement for insurance examinations, employment physicals, and the like, for they wish to present the patient in as favorable a light as possible. Reports of values obtained in this way may tend to underestimate blood-pressure levels (Society of Actuaries, 1959).

The circumstances under which the blood pressure is measured are a prime factor to be included in a definition of hypertension. In the Framingham Study the procedure called for several measurements; initially by a nurse, then two determinations by the examining physician—one at the beginning of the physical examination and a second at completion. The first determination by the clinic physician was considered most comparable to that obtained by the family physician and has been the one most frequently used in our analyses.

The blood pressures were taken with the patient in a sitting position, the left arm resting on the examiner's desk. The hour of the examination was not designated, although in retrospect this would have been desirable information. Clearly, to obtain the most comparable figures on the same patient the measurements should be repeated at the same time of day. Usually at least an hour had elapsed since the patient had eaten. Some subjects had consumed alcohol or smoked tobacco, but not in the previous hour. The systolic level was recorded at the first appearance of sound as the pressure was lowered, the diastolic at the disappearance of sound. If the sound persisted as the cuff pressure was continually lowered, the point of change from loud to soft was used.

We now believe that the decision to define blood-pressure categories prior to making any measurements was unwise. There is no doubt that the examiners were influenced in their recording by prior knowledge of these categories. If the measurements obtained were close to the limits of normal and borderline or borderline and hypertensive, the examiners tended to report a lower figure than they might have if no prior categories had been established. This is evident from the grouping of blood-pressure readings at the break points of the categories. Physicians have been conservative in their reporting of pressures for many years. Antihypertensive treatment carries some risk to the patient, so that physicians do not wish to treat anyone who does not have a real abnormality.

From mortality experience there was evidence to suggest that a rough classification into normotension, hypertension, and borderline using the following definitions would be valuable in the prognosis of this disorder (WHO, 1959):

Normotension—both pressures recorded by the physician are less than 140/90 mm Hg;

Hypertension—both pressures recorded by the physician are 160/95 and above;

Borderline—all pressures recorded are above 139/89 but below 160/95.

This classification was generally acceptable and therefore was utilized in the Framingham Study. Although of working value to the medical practitioner, any such classification clearly has the disadvantage of all attempts to convert continuous variables into qualitative categories. Since a rise of only a few millimeters of mercury, either systolic or diastolic, may change a subject's classification, considerable misclassification can occur on successive measurements. A review of the readings made at two-year intervals on randomly selected subjects indicates that although there was frequently a variation in classification at different examinations between normal and borderline or between borderline and abnormal, rarely was a person classified as hypertensive at one examination and found to be normotensive at another, or vice versa.

METHODS FOR RECORDING BLOOD PRESSURE MORE OBJECTIVELY

Blood pressure was measured in the Framingham Study by the time-honored mercury manometer. Attempts have been made for some time to correct for human error in blood-pressure determination. One such method changes the baseline from zero to a number not known to the examiner until completion of the reading (Rose, Holland, and Crowley, 1964). I have had considerable experience with this "Zero Muddler" and feel that the alleged improvement in accuracy is not achieved. Another approach, which offers considerable promise, eliminates the human ear by electronically recording the pressure. Comparison of the values obtained by such a device with those measured in the usual manner suggests that it may soon be possible to eliminate human error by truly objective electronic devices. Whether they are of sufficient benefit to warrant the cost is questionable unless the examiner has a hearing defect that interferes with determining the Korotkoff sounds.

Because repeated blood-pressure determinations on the same person vary so much, there are those who are convinced that there must be a considerable measurement error. This inference is made primarily by statisticians, who are accustomed to the measurement of variables that have fixed values about which repeated observations fluctuate. Biostatisticians are presumably more familiar with this problem, but even they have difficulty appreciating the fact that the blood pressure of a given person is not fixed. The question of which set of numbers best describes the blood pressure of a given individual is still undetermined. Many physicians seek to ascertain the lowest value of an unspecified set of measurements, with the number of readings determined by the examiner's conviction that further repetitions will not yield a lower figure. Others prefer baseline blood pressure (Smirk, 1957), measured after removal of all stimuli that might elevate the blood pressure. Determinations are usually made in a deep sleep, which has been induced by sedation. There is obvious interest in noting how low a person's blood pressure may go under such circumstances. If a subject with hypertension develops a marked drop in pressure when measured at baseline, there is reason to believe that either a surgical sympathectomy as done some years ago or a present-day "medical sympathectomy" will be extremely effective.

If our objective in measuring blood pressure is aimed at determining the status over a 24-hour period, or the *usual* pressure, then it is more likely that a casual pressure, or preferably the average of several casual pressures, will best reflect the situation. Determination of the highest or the lowest pressure, while certainly helpful in describing the blood-pressure characteristics of a given individual, may have minimal value if such pressures are in effect for only brief periods of time. Severe hard work or exercise, as we have said, may result in high systolic pressure during the period of exertion. Levine suspected years ago that such activity might be deleterious to the cardiovascular system because of the high systolic blood pressure observed in athletes while performing strenuous exercise (Levine and Brown, 1929). The fact that such exertion is only for short intervals may minimize any such hazard. Unless the very temporary blood-pressure elevation produces immediate damage—such as a ruptured vessel—the long-term harm may be negligible and is probably more than compensated by the benefit of exercise on metabolism and weight.

Casual blood pressure as determined in the usual physical examination, although apparently the least sophisticated of the measurements, may be the most satisfactory in terms of estimating the usual level. Several such determinations taken over a 24-hour period are ideal and best reflect the usual pressure. When electronic devices are perfected, it may become practicable to measure pressures frequently for a day or more and thus obtain an accurate record of blood-pressure behavior. Until that time, repeated casual pressures appear to give the best estimate.

The decision to use casual pressures in the Framingham Study was largely motivated by practicability; in an ambulatory population little else was readily obtainable. It was apparent that data based on measurements that could not readily be made in a clinical situation were unlikely to prove of practicable value. Although it was agreed that several blood-pressure measurements made at more than one examination period might be desirable, we eventually decided to obtain three determinations at one examination.

Beginning with the initial examination of the study population in 1950, blood-pressure measurements of each subject were made in an identical manner at subsequent biennial examinations. Except for occasional missed examinations, which fortunately were few, these measurements have been repeated for a 24-year period (13 biennial examinations). Since some of the subjects died or did not return for examination, the same identical cohort was not seen at each cycle. However, we can still draw some conclusions by looking at the data in several ways: for all persons who were available for any examination; for only those persons who completed all examinations; for only those persons who reported for the final examination; or for other specific groups.

Blood Pressure at the Initial Examination

Both the systolic and diastolic blood-pressure curves follow a normal or Gaussian pattern, with skewing to the right indicating that there are some subjects with pressures higher than would occur if they were strictly "normal" (as is the case with height). The same phenomenon may also be observed in many biological variables subject to environmental influences.

Several questions are immediately raised by these distribution curves. Why has skewing occurred? Why does the blood pressure not distribute purely as a normal characteristic? Why, even without the skewing, is there such a wide range of blood pressure in a presumably healthy population, essentially free of cardiovascular disease? If it were possible to remove certain subjects who contributed to the skewing of the curve, would the remainder be free of hypertension in spite of any blood-pressure elevation? Are there possibly some people with elevated blood pressure who have normal or benign hypertension? We may ask whether the average blood pressure of this population is the most desirable, or whether the ideal pressure is represented by the lowest or some intermediate point on the curve. Above all, we wish to know what contributes to the wide distribution of blood pressure and, assuming that some levels are more desirable than others, what contributes to the presence or development of the less desirable pressures. In short, we want to understand the epidemiology of blood pressure.

Refinements of the blood-pressure distribution should throw some light on this subject. Since the age and sex of the participants may make a difference, we need to look at the distribution curves for more homogeneous groups with respect to these characteristics. Such curves differ somewhat from the curve for the entire population but still maintain the basic configuration. A comparison of the 30-year-old subjects with those age 59 may be expected to show the effect of aging on blood-pressure level. That these represent different cohorts and that factors other than aging have been affecting these populations must be kept in mind.

AGE AND BLOOD PRESSURE

A review of the data from the initial examination indicates unequivocally that aging or factors associated with it affected the blood-pressure level, which rose with age. At any age and in either sex there was a wide range of blood-pressure levels. However, age and sex, in this population of adult Americans, gave only a partial explanation of the blood-pressure distribution.

The increase with age was greater in women than in men. In the age group 35-39, the average blood pressure at initial examination was 122/78 for the women compared to 132/83 for the men. In the 55-59 age group, the reverse was the case (150/90 for women compared to 140/87 for men). In the age group 45-49, blood pressures were almost identical in both sexes. Still looking at the blood-pressure distribution curves from the first examination, we may ask several more questions—one in particular: Are there other characteristics that appear to relate to blood-pressure level? The answer may be found by examining the characteristics of subjects at either end of the distribution curve.

A review of these characteristics suggests that only one factor, weight,* made any important contribution to blood-pressure level as measured in this cross section of the population (Fig. 6-1). In spite of repeated attempts to find other relevant factors, we have been unable to explain the large differences in blood pressure observed in the general public. Although we did not perform all the possible examinations some might wish, such as psychiatric evaluation, we did look at many items (including salt intake) on a study population subsample (Dawber et al., 1967). The hypothesis that sodium intake is responsible for elevation of blood pressure has always been most intriguing, but no relation of salt intake to blood-pressure level was observed. Our study did not include persons with the extremely low intakes of sodium necessary to lower blood pressure in patients with evident hypertension. The absence of sufficiently low intakes may have precluded the possibility of demonstrating a relationship of sodium intake to blood-pressure level.

Longitudinal Measurement of Blood Pressure

The plan of the Framingham Study included a long-term (20 or more years) follow-up of its population, which would provide not only an opportunity to relate a given characteristic to disease development, but also to observe any longitudinal changes in the characteristic. Observations of the effect of age on blood-pressure levels made in a cross section of the popula-

---

*Relative weight was determined by comparing the weight of the individual to the median for the age and sex group applicable.

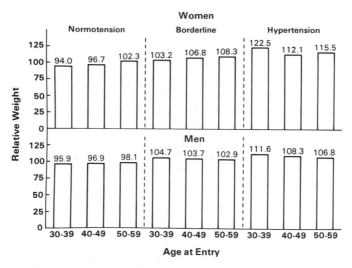

Fig. 6-1 *Relative weight, by blood-pressure category.*

tion must take into account that they are recorded at different ages in different people. Each age group must be considered a separate cohort exposed to certain variations in environment and way of life. The fact that the oldest decade (50-59) had higher blood pressures than the youngest (30-39) may represent only the effect of age, but may also reflect exposure to infections and chemical agents, nutritional habits, and/or many other variables.

Longitudinal observations of blood-pressure level in the *same* individuals provide a better opportunity to determine the effects of aging. All things being equal, we would expect the changes that occur in the same individuals as they grow older to resemble those observed cross-sectionally in the population made up of different age groups. If some factors of host or environment are affecting blood pressure (treatment for hypertension, for instance) the trend toward a rise with age may be changed.

One of our most interesting observations is the drop in blood pressure that occurred during the first four years. At the initial examination the mean systolic and diastolic pressures were greater than those observed on the second examination, which in turn were higher than those observed on the third examination (Table 6-1). From then on, the blood pressure rose consistently with age. For men the rise observed cross-sectionally was

Table 6-1 Mean blood-pressure levels of the total Framingham Study population. Only subjects who took both exam 3 and exam 13 are included.

Exam no.	Blood pressure	
	Systolic (mm Hg)	Diastolic (mm Hg)
1	131.7	83.1
2	128.6	80.7
3	127.0	79.9
4	129.7	81.4
5	130.8	81.7
6	133.0	83.0
7	134.5	83.7
8	135.8	82.3
9	137.3	81.8
10	137.8	80.6
11	—	—
12	142.0	82.1
13	139.9	79.4

matched by a similar rise longitudinally. When blood-pressure levels of women were similarly examined, the rise was less steep than that observed some 20 years ago. Instead of rising above that of men at approximately age 45, Fig. 6-2 shows that blood pressure in women measured longitudinally never reached the level of that of the male population.

We have seen that body weight is the only factor that appears to be important in relation to blood-pressure level. If we compare weight gain of subjects to changes in blood pressure, we find that gain alone does not account for the rise in blood pressure with age. One factor that might account for the diminished blood-pressure rise with age longitudinally is the use of antihypertensive therapy, which some of the subjects had been receiving.

ANTIHYPERTENSIVE THERAPY

At the time the Framingham Study began, therapy for hypertension was in its infancy. For the most part it consisted in minimal barbiturate sedation and weight control. The difficulties of the rice/fruit diet and other sodium-free regimens made such

OBSERVATIONS ON BLOOD-PRESSURE MEASUREMENT

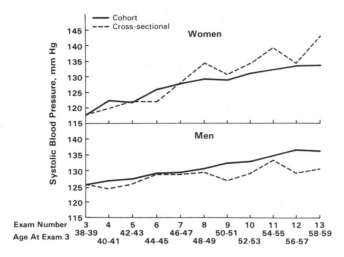

Fig. 6-2 *Trends of systolic blood pressure for cross-sectional and cohort data (subjects age 38-59 at exam 3).*

treatment essentially impossible except for a very few (usually those who had advanced hypertension, often with severe complications such as congestive failure). During the course of the study the various agents used today to treat elevated blood pressure were gradually introduced. Reports of the physical status of the Framingham subjects, including blood-pressure values, were supplied to family physicians with attention directed to any change of status; it would therefore be expected that the participants would not only be placed on antihypertensive treatment but would very likely receive much more therapy than a similar group not so carefully evaluated.

A comparison of the blood pressure determined cross-sectionally at the third examination (when blood pressures reached their lowest point) with the longitudinal observations is presented in Fig. 6-2. It is apparent that the blood pressure rise with age in men is greater when measured longitudinally than cross-sectionally at the time of the third examination. In women, however, the longitudinal observations show a less steep rise with age and never exceed those of the men. This also holds true for subjects who were at any time placed on antihypertensive medication as well as those who never used such drugs (Fig. 6-3). In subjects age 38-39 at the beginning of observation, a drop in pressure in the treated group after the tenth examination

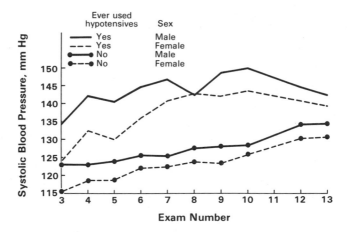

Fig. 6-3 *Trends of systolic blood pressure, by treatment status, in subjects age 38-39 at exam 3.*

occurred in both men and women. The failure of this effect to be manifest when the entire population was included may have resulted from the smaller percentage of male hypertensives receiving treatment.

From Fig. 6-3 it is apparent that antihypertensive treatment may have been a factor affecting the rise of blood pressure with age, at least in women. The effect on blood pressure in men was less convincing. Antihypertensive therapy may in fact have had little effect in controlling the blood pressure in the total male cohort. The fact that there was a drop in pressure in the men receiving antihypertensive therapy, although not as impressive as in the women, suggests two major possibilities: (1) women were more conscientious than men, both in seeking medical attention and in following the recommendations made; (2) antihypertensive therapy is more effective in women than men. There is evidence that the first of these possibilities is valid. Whereas 30 percent of the women with hypertension gave a history of being on antihypertensive medication, only 15 percent of the men similarly diagnosed admitted to taking therapy. Similarly, a higher percentage of women reported being under medical care for any reason. The second possibility, that antihypertensive treatment is not as effective in men as in women, is supported by Fig. 6-3. The data there suggest that for the last six years of observation antihypertensive treatment had an important effect in reversing the upward trend in blood pressure with age for men as well as women. The average blood pressure achieved for men was, however, still higher than that for women.

Another important conclusion that can be drawn from Fig. 6-3 is that the previously observed steeper rise in blood pressure with age in women compared to men was no longer true even in those *not* receiving antihypertensive therapy. The lessened rise in blood pressure with age in women may therefore represent some basic change in the natural history of hypertension we do not yet understand.

Certain other questions can be explored from the longitudinal data, for instance whether the rate of rise in blood pressure is a function of initial blood pressure. It has long been believed that those persons who have rather low blood pressure are less inclined to develop hypertension. This may be related at least in part to the artifact of defining hypertension in terms of absolute blood-pressure measurement. If there is a rise in blood pressure with age, and if those who pass a selected upper level of normal are declared to have developed hypertension, clearly the closer to that line the blood pressure is the more likely it will cross into the hypertensive category. Given the same degree of rise in blood pressure with age, the person with a systolic measurement of 150 mm Hg is far more likely to develop so-called hypertension than the person with a reading of 120 mm Hg.

If we compare the experience of persons in the lowest with those in the highest decile of systolic blood pressure, we fail to observe any important difference in the rate of rise with age. It would appear, then, that the initial blood pressure is important in determining whether the subject will develop hypertension— not because of any difference in tendency for the pressure to rise, but rather because the lower it is the more it must rise before it reaches the arbitrary cut-off point categorized as hypertension.

In summary, although valuable pieces of information regarding the epidemiology of elevated blood pressure were obtained from the Framingham Study, our original goal was not achieved. We had hoped to determine what causes the blood pressure of some individuals to rise to a height that appears to be dangerous, while others maintain levels only slightly higher than ob-

served in their youth. The only environmental factor of importance in elevating blood pressure was weight gain. Obviously,
there was great variability in blood-pressure level. The distribution curve was skewed to the right, with more persons demonstrating higher than expected pressures. There was also a shift
to the right with age. The rise was similar regardless of the initial pressure. The reason why persons in the upper ranges of
normal or borderline pressures develop more hypertension appears to be their increased risk of reaching the cut-off point because of their proximity to it, rather than any tendency for their
pressures to rise at a more rapid rate.

Hypertension as a Risk Factor

7

ALTHOUGH WE ARE a long way from determining the factors that lead to elevation of blood pressure in a given individual, we can nevertheless use this characteristic in studying the atherosclerotic diseases—the major problem in cardiovascular disorders. The data in the previous chapter indicate that the mean systolic and diastolic blood pressures of the population rise with age, whether studied cross-sectionally or longitudinally. This rise is relatively slight and accounts for only a small part of the explanation for the occurrence of hypertension. Very clearly, certain individuals develop a rise in blood pressure substantially above what might be expected from age alone. For the vast majority, however, the blood pressure measured during early adulthood is a reliable index of that which will prevail over the adult years. Persons who have developed unduly high levels may be separated into two groups: (1) those whose pressures were relatively high at a younger age and rose with age at the usual rate, attaining levels considered hypertensive; and (2) those whose early blood pressure was not in the upper range, but rose at a steeper gradient to reach hypertensive levels.

I have suggested that the casual pressure best characterizes the usual blood-pressure status—that is, the average pressure operating over a 24-hour period. I have also indicated that it is a reliable characteristic in terms of reproducibility. Since the original casual pressure reasonably well describes the individual, it can be used as a characteristic against which to determine the risk of the subsequent development of blood-pressure-related disorders.

The importance of elevated blood pressure in mortality and morbidity from certain disorders has been recognized for many years. Insurance-company data, used to calculate longevity, have attested to the added risk of earlier death when markedly elevated pressures are present. The medical profession too has recognized the importance of blood-pressure measurement, but has been more inclined to use the determination as a signal to look for a number of diseases related to hypertension. If these cannot be found, the typical practice has been to label any blood-pressure elevation, unless extremely high, as benign— indicating watchful waiting.

At the time the Framingham Study was designed, it was recognized that elevated blood pressure was common in patients dying of atherosclerotic diseases. The prevalence of hypertension appeared to be higher than would be expected in the general population. Hypertension led to earlier and more severe atherosclerosis of the coronary artery. The pressures referred to were relatively high and in persons who were at the extreme upper end of the distribution curve (Allan, 1934; Master, Marks, and Dack, 1943; Perera, 1948).

The difficulty of determining the relation of a number of characteristics to either the prevalence or the incidence of disease, unless measurements can be made in the general population, has prevented adequate knowledge of the epidemiology of some diseases that have a long natural history. The practicing physician may find it impractical to conduct epidemiologic studies on his own patients; he cannot be certain how representative they are of the general population, and he has no disease-free cohort with which to compare them (Liebow, Hellerstein, and Miller, 1955). In fact, he can be sure that his population is *not* representative in that it contains much larger numbers of subjects with an already diagnosable disease. He has trouble obtaining a sufficiently large comparative group of subjects who have no disorder and no need to seek medical care. In spite of widespread efforts urging everyone to obtain periodic physical checkups, very few healthy adults in the United States do so.

Patients who seek medical attention are much more likely to have severe manifestations of any disease. In the past those with elevated blood pressure have not sought medical attention until and unless complications or associated illness have caused them to do so. That physicians of previous generations were inclined to consider hypertension a manifestation of a disease process, such as renal disease, and to label the elevated blood pressure as benign when no associated disorder could be found, is understandable. Because there were no reliable data on the prevalence of hypertension in the well population, the common finding of elevated blood pressure in coronary heart disease could not be satisfactorily interpreted.

By attempting to enlist all available individuals in the population regardless of need for or interest in medical care, the Framingham Study and similar enterprises hoped to be able to evaluate the importance of a number of human characteristics —measurable long before any disease was apparent—to the eventual development of atherosclerotic disease. The original objective was confined to coronary heart disease but was later enlarged to consider the other atherosclerotic diseases and congestive heart failure as well.

The selection of a hypothesis relating blood-pressure level to cardiovascular disease was natural and reasonable in view of already published data from insurance statistics and from the experiences of a number of physicians. It was logical to assume that the greater the pressure against the arterial walls, the more likely that they would rupture or that mechanical damage which might lead to atherosclerotic changes would occur. It was also reasonable to believe that the heart that had to pump blood against an increased pressure would fail much earlier than if the pressure were lower.

Convincing evidence of the importance of blood-pressure elevation in the direct production of atheromatous lesions was the virtual absence of any such changes in the pulmonary arterial system. The pressure in this circuit was always much lower than the lowest systemic arterial pressures, unless raised by congenital or acquired diseases obstructing pulmonary blood flow— such as mitral stenosis or congenital pulmonic stenosis. The level of blood pressure tolerable in the systemic system without development of atherosclerotic changes was unknown.

Several theories to account for the role of blood pressure in atherosclerosis have been considered. A direct pressure effect might damage the intimal cells, leading to earlier deposition of atheromatous material. The pressure in the arterial lumen might affect the rate of filtration of cholesterol into the intimal arterial cells (if that is the process that actually takes place). Repeated stretching of the arterial walls via a wide pulse pressure might damage the intima. And it has been suggested that the loss of elastic tissue in the arterial wall might be one of the earlier changes in the atherosclerotic process (Dawber, Thomas, and McNamara, 1973).

Relation of Blood Pressure to Coronary Heart Disease

Examination of the relation of blood-pressure level to development of coronary heart disease was first possible after four years of follow-up (Dawber, Moore, and Mann, 1957). At that time the number of subjects who had developed coronary heart disease was minimal, so only limited observations could be made. Very little disease had as yet occurred in the younger cohort of the population. However, in the older men (age 45-62 at the beginning of the study) there was a distinctly higher rate of coronary heart disease in those classified as hypertensive (98 per 1,000) than in those classified as normotensive (26 per 1,000). As larger numbers of subjects moved into the coronary heart disease category, subsequent analyses supported the original finding. A more definitive classification of elevated blood pressure became possible, as well as estimation of risk according to systolic pressure, diastolic pressure, and various combinations of these. Determination of risk on the basis of blood pressure measured in much younger individuals, both men and women, also became feasible.

Utilizing all the data collected over the 24 years of the study, let us first look at the risk of subsequent coronary heart disease relative to blood pressure measured at initial examination. The importance of blood-pressure level to the development of atherosclerotic diseases will be readily apparent. The different manifestations of these disorders will be considered separately and analyzed in terms of the various methods of classifying blood pressure.

Coronary Heart Disease According to Blood-Pressure Categories

Coronary heart disease, as we have seen, includes several clinical entities: angina pectoris, myocardial infarction, coronary insufficiency, sudden death, and death other than sudden. In the original planning of the Framingham Study it was hoped that eventually the various entities could be analyzed individually. However, during the first few years of observation we were obliged to use the all-inclusive category "coronary heart disease" because of insufficient numbers in the individual clinical entities.

When blood-pressure level is evaluated in terms of coronary heart disease development, a strong relationship is apparent. Using the categorization of normotension, borderline, and hypertension for both men and women regardless of age at entry into the study, the incidence of coronary heart disease goes up from normotensive to borderline to hypertensive (Fig. 7-1). Although this classification on the basis of a single casual blood pressure taken under the usual conditions of an office visit may appear rather crude and unreliable, nevertheless the data clearly indicate the predictive importance of such a measurement. In the younger men followed for 24 years the risk of developing coronary heart disease in the hypertensive group was more than twice that of the normotensive subjects. In the older subjects the risk was somewhat less. In women the ratios were greater: although the *absolute* risk was much lower, the *relative* risk was higher. When the different clinical entities that comprise coronary heart disease are similarly analyzed, the relation of blood-pressure category to each becomes evident.

The 24-year incidence rates for myocardial infarction and angina pectoris are presented in Figs. 7-2 and 7-3. The small number of subjects in the hypertensive category in the younger age groups may explain the discrepancy in the trend. The similarity of the relation of blood-pressure category to subsequent development of myocardial infarction was readily apparent; the correlation with angina pectoris was less impressive.

The above analysis does not take into consideration any changes that may have taken place in the blood pressure of the subjects over the 24-year period. One way to evaluate this effect is to use the blood-pressure measurement closest in time *prior to the event*—measured at the last examination before the clinical appearance of disease. When we did this, the relation of blood pressure to incidence of coronary heart disease, stroke, and myocardial infarction became even more striking (Fig. 7-4). The incidence rates for the entire age period were strongly correlated with blood-pressure category. In each of the age groups the ratios remained similar, with the incidence rate among hypertensive subjects three to four times higher than among normotensives.

A possible explanation of the greater risk demonstrated by the latter analysis is that over the 24-year period the blood pressure of some of the subjects had risen considerably, placing them in higher categories. If this added pressure has a short-term effect on the appearance of clinical disease, analyses that reflect the rise in pressure will be more sensitive than those based on a measurement made many years earlier. We are hopeful that this is the explanation, for it suggests that the reverse would also be true—after the blood-pressure drop has been attained, the incidence should decrease rather rapidly. Studies are currently under way to determine the prognosis for hypertensive patients who have achieved a satisfactory drop in blood pressure.

Since the determination of the three blood-pressure categories involves consideration of both systolic and diastolic pressure, either or both of which may be elevated, some criticism of the classification may be justified. Analysis of the relationship according to systolic and diastolic pressure independently appears warranted.

Systolic Blood Pressure and Coronary Heart Disease

Among members of the medical profession there has always been a belief that the diastolic measurement was a better indicator of the degree of elevation of blood pressure, and that the systolic figure was to a great extent a measure of the relative elasticity of the arterial bed. According to this concept, we should direct our attention to the diastolic pressure with little or no concern about the systolic level. If the arterial system becomes relatively inelastic because of medial calcification (Monckeberg's sclerosis) the patient, often elderly, develops high systolic pressure with little or no change in diastolic level. This type of elevated blood pressure has been considered relatively benign.

Elevated systolic pressure in the absence of any important rise in diastolic pressure tends to be characteristic of the very elderly, in whom it has been considered largely a result of the aging process. Since an individual must perforce survive to a rather ripe age in order to develop this pattern of blood pressure, an artifact of benignity is produced: you have to survive to develop it. Many physicians still believe that this "physiologic" elevation of systolic pressure may be necessary to ensure adequate blood flow. Actually, in the general population the number of individuals with very high systolic pressure without diastolic hypertension is relatively low. Out of the entire population of 5,127 subjects accepted into the Framingham Study there were only 9 in whom the systolic blood pressure was above 180 mm Hg and the diastolic below 90. For the entire population there was a good correlation between systolic and diastolic pressures.

If the classification of blood pressure is based solely on the systolic reading without regard to the diastolic, a larger number of categories can be established. For purposes of analysis, break points of < 120, 120-139, 140-159, 160-179, and 180+ mm Hg were used, since enough subjects were thereby provided in each category for satisfactory evaluation. With this set of break points the relation of systolic blood pressure taken at initial examination to the development of coronary heart disease was much more striking than when the categories of normotension, borderline, and hypertension were used (Fig. 7-5). The gradient appeared steeper for the younger men, rising to six times the rate from the lowest to the highest blood-pressure category. This probably reflects the relatively longer period of exposure to elevated blood pressure in men observed to have systolic hypertension at an earlier age.

Not only did the risk of developing coronary heart disease increase with higher systolic blood pressure but, as might be expected, the disease appeared at a younger age (Table 7-1). This difference in the age of onset—approximately two years—may appear small, but in terms of life expectancy it is considerable. The differences in women were negligible except in the older age group where a similar trend was apparent.

Analysis of systolic blood pressure in terms of development

Table 7-1   Average age of onset of coronary heart disease, by systolic blood pressure.

Systolic blood pressure (mm Hg)	Age cohort of men			Age cohort of women
	30-39	40-49	50-59	50-59
< 120	51.1	60.0	66.5	71.1
160+	48.9	55.9	64.1	67.3

of the several clinical disorders constituting coronary heart disease showed a similar relationship (Figs. 7-6 and 7-7). The incidence rates of both myocardial infarction and angina pectoris rose significantly with increasing increments of systolic blood pressure. The relation of systolic pressure to angina pectoris was much more apparent here than when cruder blood-pressure categories were used. The extremely low rates of myocardial infarction in women with systolic blood pressures below 120 was quite remarkable (see Fig. 7-6). In fact, only 7 of these 650 women age 30-59 developed myocardial infarction over the 24 years of observation. In the lower range of the distribution curve, blood pressure seems to have had a minimal effect on the development of coronary artery disease. Although we do not have sufficient data to conclude what the critical level of systolic pressure may be (below which *no* disease would occur), persons who have readings of less than 100 mm Hg in all probability will develop extremely little coronary heart disease.

The third manifestation of coronary heart disease in which there were sufficient numbers of subjects to permit analysis was sudden death. When its incidence was analyzed in terms of blood-pressure category, it was apparent that again there was a significant correlation (Fig. 7-8). Although similar trends were suggested when the systolic pressure alone was evaluated, there were not enough subjects to permit adequate analysis with the blood-pressure breaks selected.

When the relationship between coronary heart disease and systolic pressure was analyzed on the basis of measurement at the last examination prior to the event, figures very comparable to those based on initial measurement were obtained (Fig. 7-9).

Again, the gradient of risk was even steeper, possibly indicating the importance of blood-pressure change over time. The similarity of the findings in both types of analysis is consistent with the observation that blood-pressure measurements made in early adulthood are accurate predictors of those taken later in life.

It is clear that, regardless of the diastolic figure, the systolic pressure was an excellent predictor of subsequent coronary heart disease and any of its clinical manifestations. Although the diastolic pressure was not considered in the above analysis, there was a good correlation between the two sets of measurements (Kannel, Gordon, and Schwartz, 1971). As already discussed, there were few subjects with high systolic levels in the presence of normal or low diastolic pressures. In fact, there were too few to permit analysis of the risk of high systolic pressure as the only manifestation of hypertension. The data should not be interpreted to conclude that those subjects who develop systolic hypertension without any rise in diastolic pressure necessarily carry the risk suggested.

(continued on page 103)

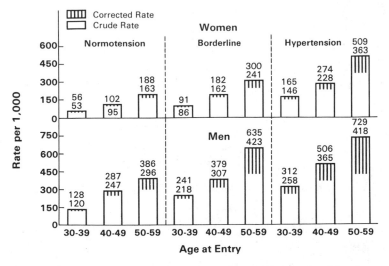

Fig. 7-1 *24-year incidence of coronary heart disease, by blood-pressure category.*

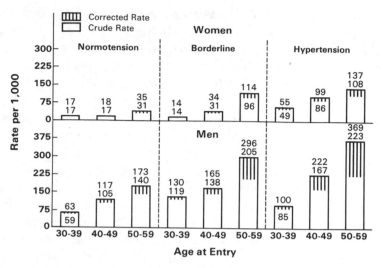

Fig. 7-2 *24-year incidence of myocardial infarction, by blood-pressure category.*

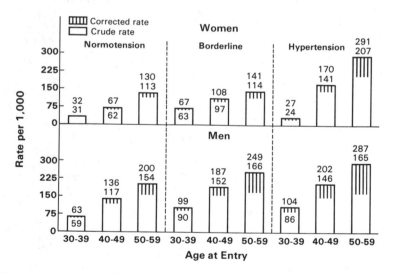

Fig. 7-3 *24-year incidence of angina pectoris, by blood-pressure category.*

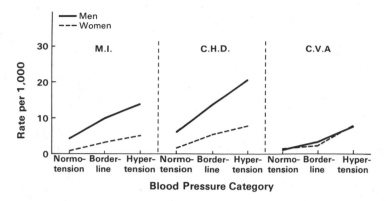

Fig. 7-4 *Average annual incidence of cardiovascular disease, by blood-pressure category. M.I. = myocardial infarction; C.H.D. = coronary heart disease; C.V.A. = cardiovascular accident.*

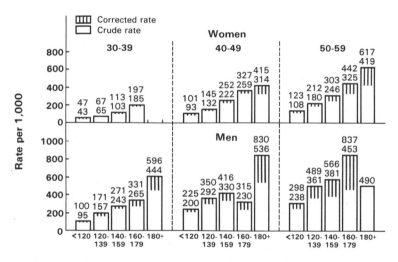

Fig. 7-5 *24-year incidence of coronary heart disease, by systolic blood pressure.*

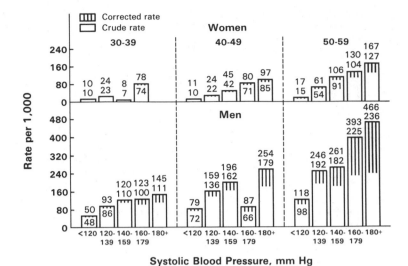

Fig. 7-6 *24-year incidence of myocardial infarction, by systolic blood pressure.*

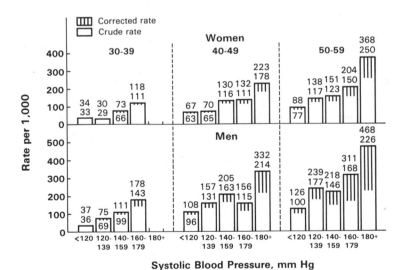

Fig. 7-7 *24-year incidence of angina pectoris, by systolic blood pressure.*

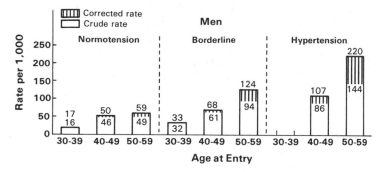

Fig. 7-8   *24-year incidence of sudden death in men, by blood-pressure category.*

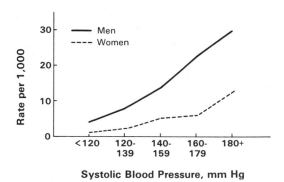

Fig. 7-9   *Average annual incidence of coronary heart disease, by systolic blood pressure.*

Diastolic Blood Pressure and Coronary Heart Disease

Classification on the basis of diastolic pressure is somewhat less precise because of the narrower range of this measurement. In the analysis presented, break points of <80, 80-89, 90-94, 95-104, and 105+ mm Hg have been used. The level of 90-94 diastolic has been considered a somewhat critical point below which the pressure was normal and above which it was abnormal—hence the selection of the 90-94 group.

The concept that slight differences in diastolic pressure have provided the distinction between normotension (below 90 mm Hg) and hypertension (95 mm Hg or greater), with a range of only 5 mm Hg (90-94) constituting borderline status, has long been accepted and is one of the bases for physicians' belief in the importance of diastolic pressure and the use of this measurement alone to determine hypertension status. In actuality the group in the narrow borderline category is sizable. Among men 30-39 years old, 9 percent were classified into the 90-94 mm Hg group, compared to 7 percent who had diastolic "hypertension." For the 40-49 age group these figures became 17 and 20 percent respectively, and for the oldest group of men 19 and 33 percent. Although the range of pressure in the borderline category is narrow, there is good reason to accept it on the basis of diastolic blood-pressure distribution. Unfortunately, because of the limited span of blood pressure in the borderline group and the difficulty of measuring diastolic pressure precisely, there is considerable opportunity for variability of classification of the same subjects on repetitive examinations.

Even though the overall relation of diastolic pressure to disease was similar to that observed with systolic pressure, it was less consistent and the gradient of increase in disease incidence was not as steep. However, essentially the same relationships were observed for total coronary heart disease and for the various clinical entities (Figs. 7-10 to 7-12). When the most recent diastolic measurement prior to the event was used, the gradient of risk of coronary heart disease was similar to that observed using the systolic pressure (Fig. 7-13). The gradient was less steep, probably owing to the difference between the distribution of the systolic and diastolic pressures. Evaluation of the other manifestations of coronary heart disease in terms of diastolic pressure was not feasible because of the limited numbers of subjects. However, the rates for sudden death were greatest in the highest diastolic blood-pressure category.

The systolic and diastolic classifications did not produce equivalent numbers of subjects in each relative category (Table 7-2). The major difference in the percentage breakdown is the larger borderline group according to systolic pressure. This has resulted in fewer subjects in the highest two systolic pressure categories. With a cut-off point of 80 mm Hg diastolic, more men were included than were found in the lowest category of systolic pressure and the rate was higher, suggesting that a lower diastolic cut-off point might be more comparable. Diastolic pressure categories can be made equivalent to those for

Table 7-2 Percentage of male subjects age 40-49 in each systolic and diastolic blood-pressure category.

Systolic blood pressure (mm Hg)	Percent	Diastolic blood pressure (mm Hg)	Percent
< 120	16.2	< 80	22.4
120-139	43.6	80-89	34.8
140-159	28.7	90-94	20.1
160-179	7.9	95-104	14.9
180+	3.6	105+	7.8

systolic pressure by creating break points of <76, 76-89, 90-99, 100-107, and 108 + mm Hg. If these break points are used and the incidence rates of myocardial infarction are compared to those determined by systolic measurement alone, the superiority of systolic pressure as a predictor still emerges (Table 7-3): in both men and women the systolic breaks determine greater differences in incidence rates of myocardial infarction than the comparable diastolic categories.

Blood pressure is an extremely important risk factor in the subsequent development of coronary heart disease. Since both systolic and diastolic pressures are important in coronary heart disease and all its clinical manifestations, it could be inferred that there would be an even greater risk of subsequent disease if both of these measurements were high. The less satisfactory performance of diastolic pressure as a predictor may be a result of the relative numbers of subjects in the upper and lower blood-pressure categories. Another reason—already alluded to—is the greater difficulty in determining the diastolic pressure precisely because of the narrower range of pressure. When a measurement cannot be readily reproduced, some misclassification is bound to occur.

Blood Pressure and Cerebral Vascular Accidents

The importance of blood-pressure level in the development of stroke has long been recognized. However, the entity "stroke" was incorrectly believed to be primarily caused by cerebral hemorrhage. The breaking of the arterial wall was logically related to the intraarterial pressure. The cardiovascular disorders

Table 7-3 Myocardial infarction by blood-pressure levels: systolic and diastolic, average annual incidence rates per 1,000.

Men (all ages)				Women (all ages)			
Systolic (mm Hg)	Incidence rate	Diastolic (mm Hg)	Incidence rate	Systolic (mm Hg)	Incidence rate	Diastolic (mm Hg)	Incidence rate
<120	3.0	<76	5.3	<120	0.7	<76	1.4
120-139	5.6	76-89	5.3	120-139	1.1	76-89	1.3
140-159	10.7	90-99	8.9	140-159	3.5	90-99	3.6
160-179	15.2	100-107	7.7	160-179	3.2	100-107	3.0
180+	18.3	108+	11.3	180+	8.6	108+	4.4

that led to embolic cerebral vascular occlusion were not necessarily blood-pressure related, and the effect of blood pressure on the production of thrombotic cerebral arterial occlusion was unknown. As pointed out earlier, although the diagnosis of the clinical event stroke is reliable, the more definitive diagnosis of the etiologic mechanism—whether it be hemorrhage, embolism, or thrombosis—is a more difficult problem even for the pathologist.

Because of the difficulties of determining with reasonable certainty the underlying basis for the clinical episode, epidemiologic studies, which have had to rely on data such as death certificates and similar reports on populations not under direct observation, have frequently been concerned with the study of stroke or cerebral vascular accidents as the only definitive end point that could be measured. In the Framingham Study we have attempted to distinguish not only stroke but also the underlying pathological basis: intracerebral hemorrhage, subarachnoid hemorrhage, cerebral embolism, or atherothrombotic brain infarction (cerebral thrombosis). However, for the benefit of those who may question the ability of the examiners to make these distinctions, the relation of blood-pressure level to the entire group of subjects developing cerebral vascular accidents is detailed herein.

An analysis of the effect of blood pressure on the development of stroke clearly indicates its importance as a risk factor. The relationship is observed in both sexes, with a similar gradient of increase in risk from normotensive to hypertensive (Fig. 7-14). Both men and women have approximately three times the probability of developing stroke during a 24-year period if they have hypertension than if they do not.

SYSTOLIC BLOOD PRESSURE AND STROKE

When the data were analyzed utilizing the five categories of systolic blood pressure, an even steeper gradient of risk of developing stroke was apparent (Fig. 7-15). There was approximately seven times the risk of developing cerebral vascular accidents in men with the highest systolic pressures compared to those with pressures below 120. In women the gradient appeared still higher, with a very low risk in those whose blood pressures were below 120. This low risk in women, for both coronary heart disease and stroke, suggests even more strongly the possibility that there is a critical level of systolic pressure in the range below 120 mm Hg.

The analyses above are based on the development of cerebral vascular accidents in terms of the blood pressure obtained at initial examination, without regard to any changes that may have occurred during the 24 years of observation. This initial blood pressure was a reasonably reliable characteristic of the individual in terms of reproducibility, not only at or near the time of the original determination but at subsequent examinations. Since blood pressure rises with age, and in a small number of individuals to a marked degree, we felt that analyses taking into account changes in the blood pressure would provide a better determination of risk.

Accordingly, when we analyze the effect of blood-pressure level utilizing measurements taken closer in time to the clinical event, we do not expect to find any important differences. An analysis utilizing reclassification of subjects on the basis of blood pressure measured within a five-year period prior to the event showed that the risk of developing stroke for the entire population separated by blood-pressure categories was approximately seven times higher in those labeled hypertensive at the examination immediately prior to the event than in those considered normotensive (Table 7-4). Using systolic measurements only, the risk was approximately nine times greater in the group of men with systolic blood pressures 180 or higher compared to

Table 7-4 Cardiovascular accidents by blood-pressure category: average annual incidence rates per 1,000 among subjects age 30-59 at entry.

Blood-pressure category[a]	Incidence rate	
	Men	Women
Normotensive	0.98	1.05
Borderline	3.20	2.17
Hypertensive	7.49	7.57

[a]As determined by the most recent blood-pressure measurement prior to the event.

those below 120 (Fig. 7-16). In women the gradient again was somewhat steeper. Clearly, systolic blood-pressure level, measured either remotely or close in time to the event, is highly predictive of the risk of developing a cerebral vascular accident. The similarity in the incidence rates of stroke in men and women is noteworthy, in contrast to the marked difference in the incidence of coronary heart disease in the two sexes.

DIASTOLIC BLOOD PRESSURE AND STROKE

When diastolic blood pressure was used as the characteristic of the examined subjects, a similar relationship to the development of stroke was observed (Fig. 7-17). The gradients of increased risk with increasing blood pressure were not as steep and the findings were not as consistent as with the use of systolic measurements. When the analysis was based on reclassification of subjects utilizing a blood-pressure measurement close to the time of the event, the gradient once again was approximately the same as when the original diastolic blood pressure was used.

Either systolic or diastolic pressure can be used to predict the development of cerebral vascular accidents, but in the Framingham Study the systolic pressure bore a closer relationship to the various degrees of risk than did the diastolic. This was evident whether the pressure used was one that had been recorded initially or closer to the clinical event and held true for both men and women in all ages studied.

BLOOD PRESSURE AND ATHEROTHROMBOTIC BRAIN INFARCTION

Of the various clinical entities included in the category of stroke, the only primary atherosclerotic disease is atherothrombotic brain infarction. In neither intracerebral nor subarachnoid hemorrhage is atherosclerosis an etiologic factor, although elevated blood pressure is clearly a strong element in development of the hemorrhage. Cerebral embolism may indirectly relate to atherosclerotic coronary disease because of embolism secondary to myocardial infarction or to atrial fibrillation. Possibly a major factor is atheromatous embolism from the subclavian-carotid system. However, for the study of atherosclerotic cerebral vascular disease, attention should be focused on strokes considered the result of brain infarction. Again, it must be stressed that the certainty with which a diagnosis of thrombosis as opposed to embolism can be made is far from absolute. There is always the possibility that material from an atheromatous plaque has been freed from the wall of an artery leading to the brain or within the brain substance, and has been carried farther in the arterial system as an embolus. The frequency with which this occurs is unknown, and there is no way to make a differential diagnosis on any clinical grounds. In subjects suffering from transient ischemic attacks, the probability of embolism is reasonably high.

When the Framingham data were analyzed using the previously listed criteria for atherothrombotic brain infarction, there was a steep gradient of risk according to blood-pressure category—just as for all cerebral vascular accidents—in all age groups (Fig. 7-18). Although the incidence rates were lower in the younger subjects, the gradient of risk according to blood-pressure category was similar to that of stroke in both men and women. In the older subjects in whom most of the thrombotic strokes occurred, there was three to four times the risk in persons previously categorized as hypertensive compared to the normotensive subjects. When systolic pressure alone was used in the analysis, a steeper gradient of risk was observed with increasing pressure (Fig. 7-19). Noteworthy was the extremely low rate of thrombotic stroke in women with systolic pressures below 120 mm Hg. Out of 651 women of all ages in this category of blood pressure, only 4 developed a thrombotic stroke during the 24 years of observation.

Again, when blood-pressure measurements closer to the event were analyzed in terms of atherothrombotic brain infarction development, essentially the same relationship was observed with an average rate for persons 180 mm Hg or above almost 30 times that observed in those with systolic pressures below 120 (Fig. 7-20). When diastolic pressure close to the event was analyzed, a similar but less steep gradient was observed. Thus the relationship of atherothrombotic brain infarction to blood-pressure level was comparable to that of all cerebral vascular accidents. Some relationship would of course be expected, since a relatively large percentage of the stroke group was made up of subjects having atherothrombotic brain infarction. To further clarify this issue, we decided to examine the relation of the non-atherosclerotic components of cerebral vascular accidents to blood-pressure level.

BLOOD PRESSURE LEVEL AND CEREBRAL EMBOLISM

If the clinical diagnosis of atherothrombotic brain infarction and cerebral embolism has been made with a reasonable degree of accuracy, there should be either no positive relation of cerebral embolism to blood-pressure level or the relation should be relatively weak because the clinical entities giving rise to embolic stroke are not of themselves markedly related to any elevation of blood pressure.

When we utilized the classification based on systolic blood pressure, there appeared to be a slight increase in risk of cerebral embolism in the higher blood-pressure categories (Table 7-5). The differences were not significant, and the analysis was plagued by small numbers of subjects with cerebral embolism. The 24-year incidence of cerebral embolism by either systolic or diastolic blood pressure showed no significant relationship. Obviously the subjects diagnosed as having developed cerebral embolism were also at risk of developing thrombotic stroke. Thus some of the subjects with "cerebral embolism" undoubtedly had thrombosis, not embolism. In view of this, it seems reasonable to conclude that no important correlation between blood-pressure level and embolism has been established.

If we examine the relation of blood-pressure level to intra-

Table 7-5   Cerebral embolism by blood-pressure category: 24-year incidence rates per 1,000 of subjects age 30-59 at entry.

Blood-pressure category	Incidence rate	Cases per population at risk
MEN		
Normotensive	0.8	8/1,013
Borderline	1.0	9/886
Hypertensive	1.4	6/422
WOMEN		
Normotensive	0.4	6/1,480
Borderline	1.4	13/907
Hypertensive	1.3	6/466

cerebral hemorrhage and subarachnoid hemorrhage together —although the number of cases is small—there is a rise in incidence with increasing blood-pressure level similar to that observed in thrombotic stroke (Table 7-6). Whatever the mechanism by which blood pressure acts to induce a thrombotic occlusion, the higher the blood-pressure level, the greater the risk of developing this disorder.

Blood-Pressure Level and Peripheral Arterial Disease

Peripheral arterial disease involving the larger arteries is first manifested clinically by intermittent claudication. The relation of blood-pressure level to peripheral arterial disease has been

Table 7-6   Cerebral hemorrhage by blood-pressure category: 24-year incidence rates per 1,000 in men and women age 30-59 at entry.

Blood-pressure category	Incidence rate	Cases per population at risk
Normotensive	8	18/2,701
Borderline	10	18/1,793
Hypertensive	17	15/888

less recognized by practicing physicians than that to stroke or coronary artery disease. In the Framingham Study, although the increase in incidence of intermittent claudication was not smooth, there was a trend in this direction using the categories of normotension, borderline, and hypertension (Fig. 7-21). With systolic pressure alone a similar trend upward with increasing pressure was present, but the trend was not consistent owing to small numbers. When the diastolic pressure was used, no significant trend was apparent. When the blood-pressure level measured closer to the event was used, a somewhat stronger relationship was apparent (Fig. 7-22). The weaker effect of blood-pressure level on peripheral arterial disease compared with stroke and coronary heart disease may result from the fact that peripheral arterial disease is more strongly related to factors (such as cigarette smoking) other than blood-pressure level.

(*continued on page 119*)

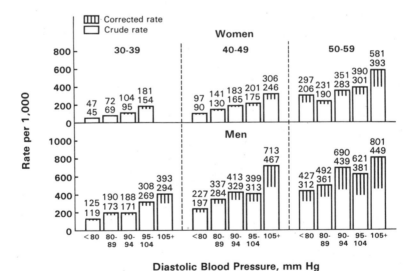

Diastolic Blood Pressure, mm Hg

Fig. 7-10 *24-year incidence of coronary heart disease, by diastolic blood pressure.*

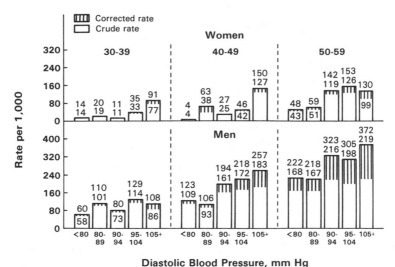

Fig. 7-11 *24-year incidence of myocardial infarction, by diastolic blood pressure.*

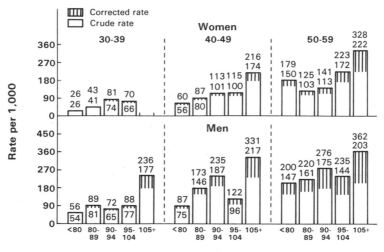

Fig. 7-12 *24-year incidence of angina pectoris, by diastolic blood pressure.*

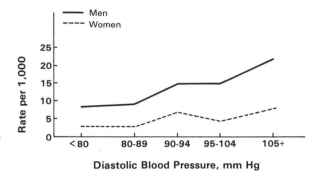

Fig. 7-13 *Average annual incidence of coronary heart disease, by diastolic blood pressure.*

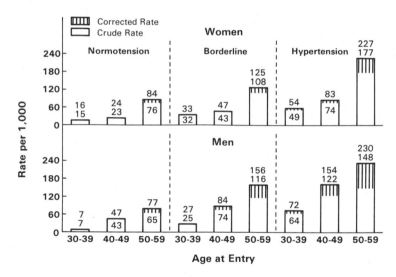

Fig. 7-14 *24-year incidence of cerebral vascular accident, by blood-pressure category.*

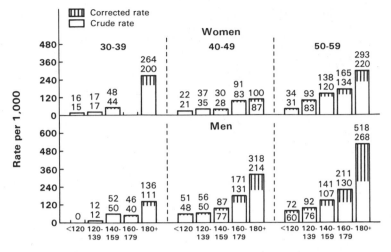

Fig. 7-15   *24-year incidence of cerebral vascular accident, by systolic blood pressure.*

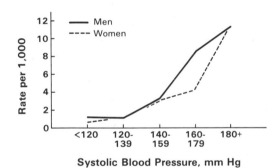

Fig. 7-16   *Average annual incidence of cerebral vascular accident, by systolic blood pressure.*

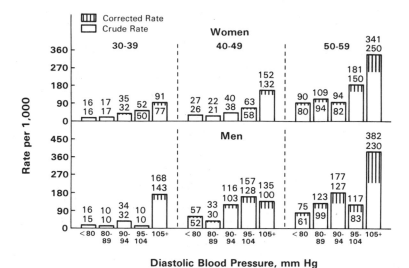

Fig. 7-17   *24-year incidence of cerebral vascular accident, by diastolic blood pressure.*

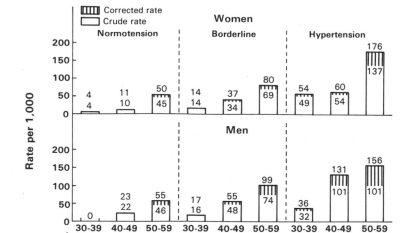

Fig. 7-18   *24-year incidence of atherothrombotic brain infarction, by blood-pressure category.*

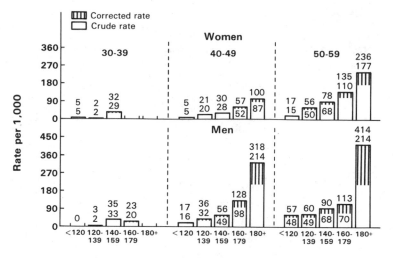

Fig. 7-19 *24-year incidence of atherothrombotic brain infarction, by systolic blood pressure.*

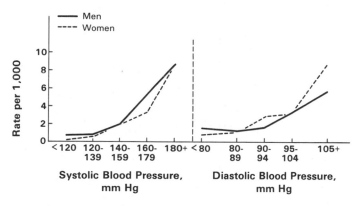

Fig. 7-20 *Average annual incidence of atherothrombotic brain infarction, by blood pressure.*

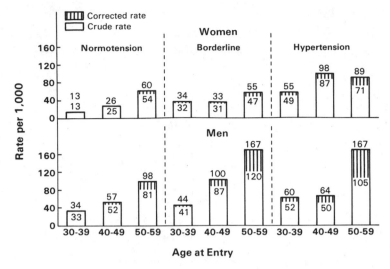

Fig. 7-21 *24-year incidence of intermittent claudication, by blood-pressure category.*

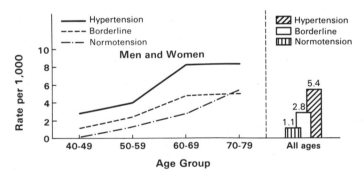

Fig. 7-22 *Average annual incidence of intermittent claudication, by blood-pressure category.*

Summary and Implications

All types of atherosclerotic disease proved to be related to blood-pressure level. The strongest relationship was seen in atherothrombotic brain infarction and coronary heart disease, with the weakest in peripheral arterial disease. The blood-pressure level, measured either years before any overt evidence of disease or close to the occurrence of the event, was strongly related to disease development. This was to be expected in view of the fact that the blood pressure of a given individual tends to remain constant over the years except for a slight rise with age. In general, the effect of blood pressure as a risk factor was greater when measured closer to the event, suggesting that blood-pressure level may be important not only in terms of accelerating the atherosclerotic process but also in precipitating the clinical event. This is an important consideration for those concerned with hypertension. It is not likely that lowering blood pressure late in atherosclerosis could have an important effect on that disorder, but it may well be beneficial in delaying the occurrence of its clinical manifestations.

The relative effect of blood pressure on the development of the atherosclerotic diseases was similar in the two sexes, although differences in the absolute risk were observed. Coronary disease was much less common in women in spite of the fact that at the beginning of this study their blood pressure after the age of 45 was significantly higher than that of men. The incidence of atherothrombotic brain infarction was similar in the two sexes and the effect of blood pressure even more pronounced in women than in men. The incidence of peripheral arterial disease is much greater in men than in women, and the correlation with blood pressure is weak in both sexes. The fact that intermittent claudication is highly related to factors such as cigarette smoking and diabetes may account for the diminished effect of blood pressure in peripheral vascular disease.

That elevated blood pressure is associated with a higher incidence of atherosclerotic diseases is clearly apparent. The benefit to be achieved by lowering blood pressure is still under study; some investigators have reported lower rates of cerebral vascular accidents in patients on antihypertensive treatment. This therapy, although it may not greatly affect atherosclerosis, may still be beneficial in curtailing overt evidence of the disease. Limited benefit may be expected in peripheral arterial disease. The mechanism by which elevation of blood pressure accelerates the atherosclerotic process is not known.

It is probably safe to assume that the length of time over which the pressure has been elevated is highly important. This factor is not taken into consideration in the usual assessment of antihypertensive therapy. Speaking for myself, it seems unreasonable to believe that lowering blood pressure that has been elevated for many years can undo the deleterious effects. If ultimate benefit is to be achieved in preventing atherosclerosis, attention must be directed toward keeping the blood pressure from rising in the first place. Meanwhile, the detection of elevated blood pressure in apparently well individuals long before any overt evidence of damage has become manifest appears highly desirable. The physician must decide on the basis of the blood-pressure level and the presence of other risk factors whether to recommend antihypertensive therapy and, if so, what the therapeutic regimen should be.

Lipids and Atherosclerotic Disease

8

THE LONG-STANDING HYPOTHESIS that blood lipids contribute to the development of atherosclerosis has been strongly supported by numerous studies, both clinical and epidemiologic. The determination by pathologists that the major constituent of the atheromatous lesion is cholesterol strengthened the concept that cholesterol in the circulating blood, through some unknown mechanism, is deposited in the arterial wall. Other changes—fibrosis and calcification—are considered inflammatory reactions to the presence of this substance. Seventy-five years ago (Marchand, 1904) simple filtration of the lipid from the blood through the intimal wall was proposed as the means by which the atheromatous lesion was produced. Later suggestions have been that the lipid in the arterial wall develops in situ, or that it is derived from the incorporation of arterial wall thrombi into the intima (Duguid, 1949). Hemorrhages from capillaries in the wall have also been suggested, as have combinations of the above mechanisms.

Many studies support the concept that the lipids in the plaques are similar to those in the blood and that blood lipids do in fact enter the arterial wall, although the exact manner of entrance remains a mystery. Experiments have shown that lesions similar to human atherosclerosis can be produced in many animals by feeding large amounts of cholesterol and fat. Changes in the host animal are usually required (thyroidectomy in the dog, for example). Direct physical trauma to the arterial wall may be necessary to produce rapid development of experimental atherosclerosis.

Observations of the early and excessive development of human atherosclerosis have been most supportive of a relationship between blood lipids and this disorder. The nature of these observations may have affected the progress of research in this field, since the examples of early human atherosclerotic disease were limited to a very few individuals who had recognizable serious disease.

Familial Hypercholesterolemia

The most common instance of the early development of atherosclerosis, often with premature occurrence of angina pectoris or myocardial infarction, was in patients with familial hypercholesterolemia, frequently with xanthomatosis. Such individuals had excessively high blood levels of cholesterol. A comparison of the blood levels of a group of persons with this disorder to those of the Framingham population indicated the unusually high cholesterol levels of the former. Also demonstrated was the infrequency in the general population of the blood cholesterol levels usually observed in familial hypercholesterolemia (Fig. 8-1). Because the blood cholesterol distribution of those with xanthomatosis is distinctly higher than that of the general population, with very little overlap, it may be concluded that only very high levels are indicative of any important underlying disorder. Some physicians still believe that only those with these extremely high levels are at particular risk and that this is because of an underlying metabolic disorder not otherwise disclosed.

Attempts to separate the various lipid fractions in the blood have been made, with the intent of defining several lipid "diseases." This approach (which has also plagued the study of hypertension) has perhaps hindered progress in assessment of the relation of blood lipid measurements to clinical atherosclerotic disease. World-wide epidemiologic studies, however, have supported the concept that the importance of blood cholesterol measurement is not primarily because such determinations detect disorders of lipid metabolism. The blood levels of cholesterol found in populations throughout the world have provided

LIPIDS AND ATHEROSCLEROTIC DISEASE

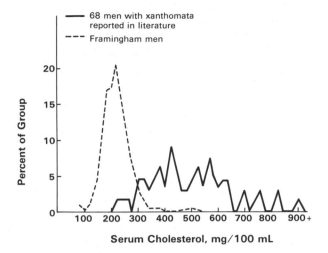

Fig. 8-1 *Distribution of serum cholesterol in men age 30-62 in the Framingham Study vs xanthomatous patients reported in the literature.*

clear evidence of the significant differences that exist among supposedly normal populations. In geographic areas where the mean of the distribution curve of blood cholesterol is considerably below that observed in the United States, there is a much lower coronary heart disease incidence. The early epidemiologic studies were perforce rather crude, a factor in the skepticism about their interpretation. Yet later, more directly clinical studies have confirmed the previous observations. The reasons for the differences in population lipid levels still have not been entirely clarified and are the subject of continuing controversy. The role of dietary fat and cholesterol in the determination of blood cholesterol levels—and thus in the development of atherosclerotic disease—still has not been defined to the satisfaction of many physicians (Mann, 1977). Others consider the evidence reasonably convincing (Stamler, 1962).

In the design of the Framingham Study it was natural that the principal hypothesis to be investigated involved the role of blood lipids, particularly cholesterol, in the development of coronary heart disease. We also wished to explore the suggestion that phospholipid values might be of importance. Accordingly, plans were made to determine these two lipid moieties at the initial examination and to repeat the determinations at the subsequent biennial examinations.

One of the problems that had plagued the study of blood cholesterol was the difficulty of obtaining accurate, repeatable measurements. The usual laboratory determinations were of value in clinical practice, which (as indicated above) was almost entirely concerned with the confirmation of excessively high levels in persons with known or suspected disease. However, the wide range of variability observed in most clinical laboratories on repeated evaluation of the same blood serum specimen was not acceptable when lesser degrees of difference in the level were to be measured in the nondiseased population. For this reason we elected to determine serum cholesterol by the Abell-Kendall method (Abell et al., 1952), which had a proven record of accuracy on repetitive determinations.

Initial experience showed that in the hands of the Framingham laboratory personnel, determinations of serum cholesterol in the usual ranges observed could be repeated with differences of no more than 10 mg %, and usually within 5 mg %. This laboratory measurement was monitored closely, including an exchange of specimens with other laboratories and with the new laboratory established by the U.S. Public Health Service at the Center for Disease Control in Atlanta. These details are mentioned because in 1950 the medical profession was exceedingly skeptical of the value of performing the test at all in view of the lack of consistent valid measurements.

Data accumulated previously demonstrated that cholesterol levels in the blood are not affected by recent ingestion of food. This made measurement practicable in an ambulatory population in whom fasting measurements would have been difficult to obtain. Blood specimens were taken at the completion of the physical examination, with the subject lying down to avoid any syncopal attack. More recent claims that cholesterol level varies with body position suggest the need for uniformity in this regard, but the importance of body position as a factor may be exaggerated.

Distribution of Cholesterol Level in the Framingham Study

From the initial measurements of serum cholesterol in the Framingham Study it was possible to describe this characteristic in a normal, or nondiseased, population. Distribution curves based on these measurements for both sexes and for different age groups are presented in Fig. 8-2. Although there was a rea-

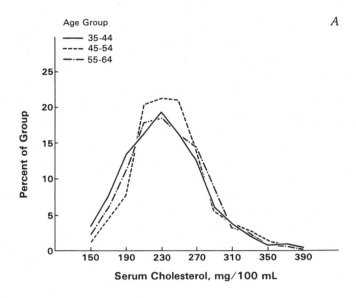

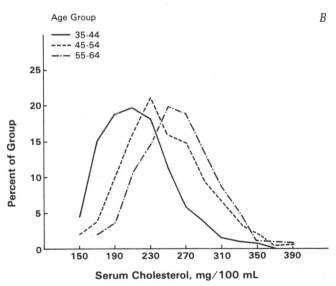

Fig. 8-2 *Distribution of serum cholesterol in 1,875 men (Fig. 8-2A) and in 2,256 women (Fig. 8-2B) in the Framingham Study.*

sonably wide range of values, almost all lay between 150 and 400 mg %. There was no double hump, no suggestion that the distribution curve was composed of two distinctly different curves representing both a normal and a diseased population. There were only a few individuals with the very high levels consistent with lipid metabolic disease. In Fig. 8-1 the distribution curve of cholesterol levels in subjects with xanthomatosis lies considerably to the right of that of the Framingham population; although some measurements lie within the Framingham range, they are distinctly unusual.

The distribution curve of blood cholesterol in the Framingham population is essentially normal, with slight skewing to the upper values. All but the very high levels observed in this curve can therefore be attributed to normal biological variability rather than to the existence of an undiagnosed metabolic disease. The few persons with exceptionally high levels are insufficient to produce marked skewing of the curve.

Other important conclusions can be reached from a study of these data. In men, aging has essentially no effect on serum cholesterol level at least over the 30-year span of adulthood studied (ages 30-59). Among the women, however, a significant rise in serum cholesterol level with age is evident. The shape of the curve was unchanged, but with increasing age the entire curve shifted to the right.

THE EPIDEMIOLOGY OF SERUM CHOLESTEROL

To describe a characteristic fully it is important to know its relation to other factors that may be involved in disease development. We need to know the epidemiology of serum cholesterol: we need to know what contributes to the presence and strength of the risk factor itself. Past observations of serum cholesterol level and its relevance to disease were concerned with the high levels of cholesterol in the blood of persons with lipid metabolic diseases. At one time it may have appeared that by identifying persons with such diseases, the relation of blood cholesterol to atherosclerotic disease would have been clarified. However, there is little evidence from the distribution curves that lipid-abnormality "disease" contributes materially to the incidence of atherosclerosis unless very large numbers of apparently healthy individuals are suffering from some hitherto unrecognized abnormality. Persistent efforts have been made to imply that such is the case. Further classification of subjects on the basis of other lipid moieties, the manner in which cholesterol is transported in the blood, and fractionation of lipoproteins has been carried out in an attempt to suggest that the apparently normal distribution of serum cholesterol masks hidden disease.

Age and Sex

The initial observations of the effect of age and sex on cholesterol level indicated no age relationship in men but an important one in women. In the middle decade (40-49 years) the curves for men and women were almost superimposable. In the 30-39 decade the women had lower levels, whereas by the 50-59 decade their levels were higher than those of men.

Cholesterol Level and Other Risk Factors

The relation of serum cholesterol level to other important risk factors has been analyzed elsewhere (Kannel et al., 1962). That report concluded that the differences in serum cholesterol in the Framingham subjects could not be accounted for by any other variables that had been measured. The interrelation of other risk factors with cholesterol level is indicated in Table 8-1.

Blood Pressure

There was a positive association between serum cholesterol level and both systolic and diastolic blood pressure. Although the differences in pressure in the several cholesterol categories were minimal, the effect over time would be a slight increase in the risk of elevated serum cholesterol on the basis of the associated blood-pressure elevation. Some of this may result from a secondary association with relative weight.

Relative Weight

Again, although the relationship of relative weight to cholesterol level was not very strong, it was positive. In the younger men the difference amounted to 6-7 percent of relative weight between the upper and lower cholesterol levels. Some of the adverse effect of elevated cholesterol in men can be attributed to this association with body weight. In women there was no consistent relationship except in the 40-49 age group. Curiously, it

Table 8-1 Correlation of cholesterol level with other risk factors.

Cholesterol level	Blood pressure		Relative weight[a]	Uric acid (mg %)	No. of cigarettes per day	Physical activity index[b]
	Systolic (mm Hg)	Diastolic (mm Hg)				
			Men			
			Age 30-39			
< 200	130	82	97	4.6	15	35
200-259	133	85	103	5.0	17	34
260+	135	86	105	5.1	18	34
			Age 40-49			
< 200	133	85	99	4.7	14	34
200-259	136	87	102	4.9	15	33
260+	142	91	105	5.0	16	33
			Age 50-59			
< 200	140	86	102	4.7	10	33
200-259	144	89	102	4.9	11	32
260+	145	89	103	4.8	12	33
			Women			
			Age 30-39			
< 200	123	78	96	3.4	8	32
200-259	125	80	99	3.6	7	32
260+	126	79	97	3.5	9	31
			Age 40-49			
< 200	132	83	100	3.6	5	31
200-259	136	85	102	3.7	5	31
260+	141	88	105	4.0	6	31
			Age 50-59			
< 200	154	93	113	4.1	3	30
200-259	152	90	109	4.1	3	30
260+	153	91	107	4.1	3	30

[a]Weight compared to the median weight for the appropriate sex and height group.
[b]Derived from the history of usual 24-hour activity (see Chapter 10 for details).

was only in this age group that serum cholesterol level was shown to be an important risk factor.

OTHER FACTORS

Even though cigarette smoking was not importantly related to serum cholesterol, a slight but consistent gradient of cigarette consumption was observed in men. Uric acid levels were also positively associated, but this relationship was not of clinical importance. The degree of physical activity reported did not affect the cholesterol level, a fact that may seem curious in view of efforts to encourage more physical activity as a means of lowering cholesterol level and preventing coronary heart disease. With the narrow range of physical activity reported in this population, the lack of apparent benefit of increased activity on cholesterol level must be interpreted with caution; in more active populations an effect might be observed.

Although some correlation was found between serum cholesterol level, weight, blood pressure, and to a lesser extent other factors, the association was weak and could only account for very minimal effects of cholesterol level on disease development. The association between dietary intake and serum cholesterol level is discussed later in this chapter. In effect, as indicated in the previous report, no conclusion can yet be reached regarding the factors responsible for differences in serum cholesterol level within populations.

Cholesterol Level and Coronary Heart Disease

The factors that contribute to the blood cholesterol level in a given individual are far from completely understood. The mechanism by which cholesterol in the blood is deposited in the intimal wall and aggregates to form an atheromatous plaque has not been established either. However, there can be no doubt about the importance of blood cholesterol in the development of atherosclerotic disease. Observations from the Framingham Study over 24 years clearly indicate that serum cholesterol plays a role in the incidence of coronary heart disease (Fig. 8-3). In each of the three decades of men, total coronary heart disease increased the higher the blood cholesterol level. In the youngest decade the relative risk in men with cholesterol levels of 260 mg % or more was over four times that of men with levels below 200. In men 40-49 years old the rise was not as steep but was consistent. This was also true for the 50-59 year old men, with a slightly diminished trend.

In men at all ages the level of blood cholesterol measured at the start of a 24-year observation period was a remarkably good predictor of the incidence of all types of coronary heart disease. The value of the measurement as a risk factor decreased with age. This may be an artifact of aging rather than a decrease in the effect of cholesterol level.

Analysis of the 24-year risk in women on the basis of cholesterol level was somewhat complicated by the changing value of this characteristic with age. As Fig. 8-3 shows, in both the youngest and oldest decade examined, no significant differences in incidence rate of coronary heart disease on the basis of cholesterol level were observed. In the middle decade (40-49 years), although the absolute coronary heart disease incidence was much lower, there was a relative increase similar in magnitude to that observed in men. As noted previously, it was in this decade that the cholesterol distribution curve in women closely resembled that in men.

When analysis was based on the determination of average annual incidence rates, taking into account any changes in serum cholesterol level that might have occurred, it is not surprising that similar findings were observed (Fig. 8-4). The average annual rate during the entire 24 years for men with cholesterol levels 260 mg % or more was twice that of those with levels below 200. The gradient of increase in rate was steepest in the younger men. In women a gradient of increasing risk with rising cholesterol level was observed in the 50-59 decade, consistent with the 24-year incidence data that followed the 40-49 year cohort through this time period.

Serum Cholesterol and Myocardial Infarction

The relation of serum cholesterol level to the development of myocardial infarction was very similar to that for total coronary heart disease (Fig. 8-5). This is not surprising, as myocardial infarction is the major clinical manifestation of coronary heart disease in men. The risk in the younger men with levels of 260 mg % or higher was approximately four times that of those with less than 200. This ratio dropped to about double in the 50-

59 age group. Analysis in terms of average annual incidence rates showed a similar relation of myocardial infarction to serum cholesterol level in men (Fig. 8-6).

In women the highest rate of myocardial infarction occurred in those with cholesterol levels 260 mg % or higher, but no gradient of risk was apparent. The small numbers of subjects developing myocardial infarction in the younger women made the analysis difficult. On the basis of average annual rates there was no consistent relationship according to cholesterol level.

CHOLESTEROL LEVEL AND ANGINA PECTORIS

In men a significant and important gradient of risk in angina pectoris occurred by serum cholesterol level (Fig. 8-7). In women the gradient was seen only in the 40-49 year age group. Insufficient numbers of subjects developing disease in the youngest decade prevented analysis.

There was a striking similarity in the incidence patterns of total coronary heart disease, myocardial infarction, and angina pectoris.

SERUM CHOLESTEROL AND SUDDEN DEATH

The relation of serum cholesterol level to the subsequent occurrence of sudden death was less impressive. In the youngest group of men and in the women the incidence was too low to permit analysis. For the two older decades of men (Fig. 8-8) no significant gradient was seen. Examination of the annual incidence rates of sudden death similarly did not show an association with cholesterol levels. For the entire age group no gradient was apparent for men. The incidence rates in women were too low to permit analysis.

The lack of association between serum cholesterol level and the incidence of sudden death suggests that factors other than the atherosclerotic process may be of major importance in this manifestation of coronary artery disease. If sudden death represented the earliest sign of coronary occlusion, which would have led to myocardial infarction, we should expect a relation to serum cholesterol level similar to that seen in myocardial infarction. Sudden death apparently is almost always caused by arrhythmia. Although this may be related to myocardial ischemia, many other factors must be operative also (cigarette smoking, for example); these may not be directly connected with the atherosclerotic process. Certainly from the evidence we cannot implicate serum cholesterol level in this disorder.

Serum Cholesterol and Atherothrombotic Brain Infarction

The relation of serum cholesterol level to atherothrombotic brain infarction in the Framingham data was always somewhat equivocal. After 24 years' observation this is still the case. Although in men the incidence rates were greatest in the group of subjects with the highest cholesterol levels, a clear-cut gradient of risk was not evident (Fig. 8-9). In women no relationship was apparent. Similarly, when the average annual incidence rates of atherothrombotic brain infarction were evaluated in terms of cholesterol level, no significant relationship was observed. We must therefore conclude that thrombotic stroke, and by inference atherosclerotic cerebral vascular disease, is not importantly related to serum cholesterol level.

Serum Cholesterol and Peripheral Arterial Disease

Comparison of the lowest and highest cholesterol categories showed significant differences, with higher risk in the highest cholesterol category (Fig. 8-10). However, no consistent gradient was observed. On the basis of average annual incidence rates there was a gradient for all men from 2.0 per thousand per year in the lowest to 4.5 in the highest cholesterol group. In women the incidence rates were too low for analysis. Although the relation of serum cholesterol level to intermittent claudication was much weaker than that of certain other factors, nevertheless there was suggestive evidence that this characteristic may play a role in peripheral arterial disease development.

(continued on page 136)

LIPIDS AND ATHEROSCLEROTIC DISEASE

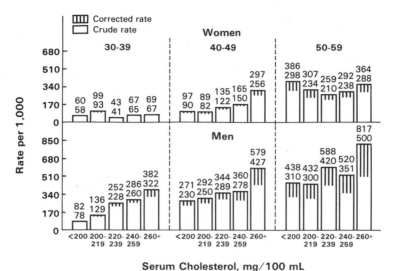

Fig. 8-3 *24-year incidence of coronary heart disease, by serum cholesterol level.*

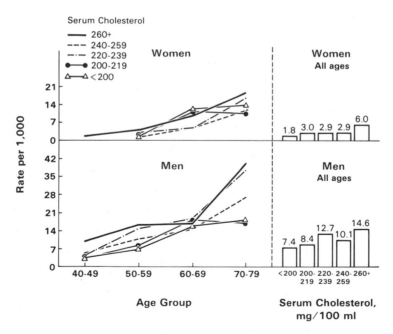

Fig. 8-4 *Average annual incidence of coronary heart disease, by serum cholesterol level.*

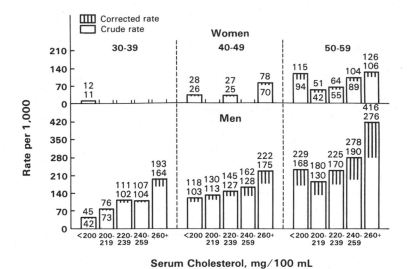

Fig. 8-5 *24-year incidence of myocardial infarction, by serum cholesterol level.*

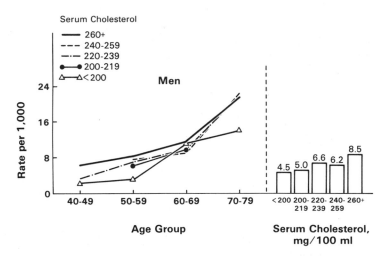

Fig. 8-6 *Average annual incidence of myocardial infarction in men, by serum cholesterol level.*

LIPIDS AND ATHEROSCLEROTIC DISEASE

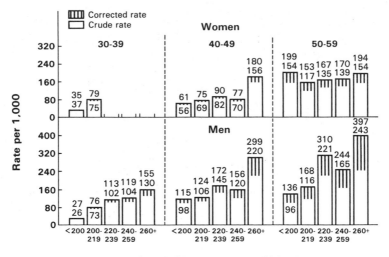

Fig. 8-7 *24-year incidence of angina pectoris, by serum cholesterol level.*

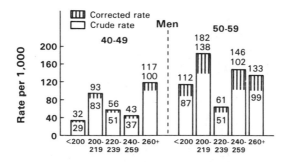

Fig. 8-8 *24-year incidence of sudden death in men, by serum cholesterol level.*

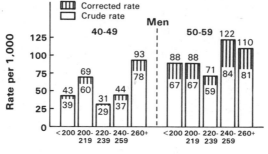

Fig. 8-9   *24-year incidence of atherothrombotic brain infarction in men, by serum cholesterol level.*

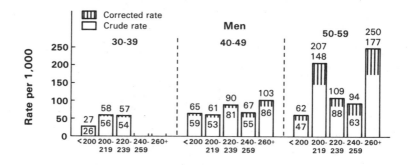

Fig. 8-10   *24-year incidence of intermittent claudication in men, by serum cholesterol level.*

Other Lipids

The initial blood lipid determinations in Framingham were limited to total cholesterol and phospholipids. The latter proved greatly inferior to the former as a predictor. Shortly after the Framingham Study was launched, the suggestion was made that the determination of certain lipoprotein moieties based on their specific gravity might be of more value than a cholesterol determination (Gofman et al., 1950). These measurements were made using an ultracentrifuge; however, the claims of superiority were disproved shortly afterward. Comparison of the relative predictability of cholesterol and ultracentrifuge measurements demonstrated that the former were of much greater value (National Advisory Heart Council, 1956).

Because the ultracentrifuge technique was difficult and expensive, its use was limited. When simpler methods of determining lipoproteins using paper electrophoresis became available, the determination of lipoproteins became practicable but with a sacrifice of the precision that could be achieved by the ultracentrifuge. It seems strange, in view of the failure to demonstrate any benefit in predictability of coronary heart disease by the Gofman technique, that so much interest has been exhibited in determining lipoprotein types by a much cruder method. Little of practical value was gained by elaborate determination of lipoprotein types, although such studies have elucidated the manner in which cholesterol is carried in the blood stream. No advantage over simple serum cholesterol determinations has been shown insofar as predictability of coronary heart disease is concerned.

Considerable interest in triglycerides has been exhibited for a number of years, but again no advantage has been demonstrated by adding this measurement beyond what might occur with repetition of the cholesterol determination itself. The more lipid measurements that are made, the more accurately the subject will be classified. If three different lipid measurements were used and all three were elevated, the subject would be at greater risk of atherosclerotic disease than if only the cholesterol level itself had been used as the criterion. However, if three cholesterol determinations were made, those subjects highest on all three would also be at greater risk than if only one determination had been used. This is a point of practical interest to the physician who wishes to determine a patient's level of cholesterolemia. Although the Framingham Study utilized only one determination at initial examination, and this measurement quite accurately classified the population, in retrospect it would have been better to have performed several tests before a classification was made. Undoubtedly if only those subjects who had serum cholesterol levels above 260 mg% on all three tests were compared with other subjects, their risk of coronary heart disease would have been still higher than that when only a single test was used.

The most recent interest has been in the possible value of determining the cholesterol in certain lipoprotein fractions and using this as a measurement of risk. Preliminary studies suggest that the level of cholesterol in the low-density lipoprotein fraction (LDL) is positively related to coronary heart disease development, while the cholesterol in the high-density lipoproteins (HDL) is negatively related (Castelli et al., 1977; Gordon et al., 1977). Combinations of these two may facilitate prediction even in the older population, in which total cholesterol level has lost predictability. Prospective studies of HDL cholesterol in young individuals have not been conducted. The value of this measurement as a predictor is unknown except in older people. From the point of view of the physician interested in prevention, this added feature would not appear to be of much importance; it is unlikely that efforts to change blood lipids at advanced age would be worthwhile.

Within the Framingham population the level of cholesterol in the blood proved to be a good predictor of the development of atherosclerotic disease. The relationship was strongest in the younger men. In women it appeared to be most important in the 40-49 year age group, for which the cholesterol distribution curve most resembled that of the men. The evidence that other lipid measurements had any benefit over cholesterol level alone is lacking, with the possible exception of the HDL cholesterol fraction.

The above data relate to intrapopulation differences. The contributing factors have not been satisfactorily determined. Other factors, such as weight and blood pressure, account for a limited amount of the variability. The expectation that the intrapopulation differences in cholesterol level could be attributed to individual dietary habits has not been fulfilled. The variability of blood cholesterol values within the Framingham population appears to reflect inherent or constitutional traits rather than differences in life habits.

The dietary intake of the subjects in the Framingham Study, and by inference of the entire United States, was quite similar (Mann et al., 1962). Regardless of economic status, the entire population was relatively well off, particularly with regard to ability to purchase food, compared with many other peoples around the world. The availability of food and the standardization of food preparation have greatly increased the uniformity of the diet. Obviously, the quantity of food reflected in body weight varied widely. However, in terms of the qualitative makeup—the percentage of calories from fat, protein, and carbohydrate; the percentage of saturated versus unsaturated fat; and the total cholesterol intake—there was limited variability. In terms of those elements of the dietary intake that are known to affect cholesterol level—total cholesterol, total fat, and the polyunsaturated-to-saturated fat ratio—essentially none of the Framingham population demonstrated sufficiently low levels of intake that any impact on blood cholesterol would be expected. None was seen. Differences of dietary intake that could affect the blood cholesterol level did not account for the intrapopulation differences nor for the effect of cholesterol level on the *relative* risk within this population.

To conclude from the Framingham data that dietary intake is of no importance in determining the cholesterol level in human populations is not justified. A considerable body of evidence has been provided from experimental studies on the effect of various diets on serum cholesterol. These studies show that the amount of fat and its composition, particularly the relative degree of saturation, together with the amount of cholesterol in the food, have an important bearing on the usual blood cholesterol level. Caloric intake is also an essential consideration. In order to achieve an important reduction in blood cholesterol it is necessary to restrict caloric intake to that required for the maintenance of optimum weight. For almost everyone this means a *decrease* in total caloric intake. Furthermore, the fat intake must be lowered so that it contributes less than 30 percent of the calories. Not only must the quantity be limited, but the quality must be changed to provide a preponderance of unsaturated fat. A ratio of two parts unsaturated to one part saturated has been recommended by the American Heart Association. At one time it was believed that the amount of cholesterol in the diet was not important; later studies, however, have indicated that a diet containing less than 200 mg per day of this substance was most effective in achieving a significant drop in the blood cholesterol level.

Not only can the level be decreased by dietary changes of the type described, it can also be elevated by a diet high in calories, especially if accompanied by decreased physical activity with consequent weight gain. Such a diet must contain a sufficient amount of fat, with a preponderance of saturated fat. High intake of cholesterol further accelerates the increase in blood cholesterol. Although some proponents of changes in dietary habits have implied that alterations necessary to achieve a drop in blood cholesterol level are relatively simple, in fact in our society persistent efforts are required to follow such routines. Minor changes, such as substituting margarine made from polyunsaturated fat for butter, will not have much, if any, effect. Merely reducing egg consumption without consideration of the total diet will have no effect. In the Framingham population, although considerable differences in eating habits were observed, these did not include the marked differences that would account for the wide range of individual cholesterol levels found.

In order to ascertain the effect of diet on cholesterol level in the Framingham Study, we must look *outside* this population and compare it to other populations living under considerably different circumstances, especially with reference to usual dietary intake. Examination of the blood cholesterol levels in many other populations throughout the world discloses considerable variability in the average values, with certain populations showing distribution curves markedly lower than those observed in the Framingham Study.

The usual dietary intake of a population has a powerful effect in determining the *average* cholesterol level. The distribution of individual values is wide, regardless of the average level. A correlation between dietary intake and intrapopulation differences has not been demonstrated when food consumption was similar. In populations where there have been marked differences of food intake, on the other hand, a relationship between blood cholesterol level and diet has been demonstrable (Keys, 1952, 1980). Even in the United States as a whole, a relationship can be found when groups following unusual dietary patterns—like the macrobiotic cult—are examined (Castelli, 1977).

Low rates of coronary heart disease in populations with low *average* levels of blood cholesterol compared with the Framingham values indicate an influence of diet on the blood cholesterol level that, in turn, affects the development of atherosclerotic disease. Within these populations differences in blood cholesterol level contribute to the *relative* risk. The intrapopulation differences must be attributed to other, possibly inherent, factors. In the Framingham population, therefore, the high average level of blood cholesterol must be ascribed to the usual American diet, high in animal fat and cholesterol, producing a high frequency of obesity and a high average risk of atherosclerotic disease.

The Framingham data provide overwhelming evidence that the level of cholesterol in the blood is a powerful factor in development of the major manifestations of coronary heart disease, myocardial infarction and angina pectoris. This evidence is so convincing that it is difficult to understand how any reasonable person could question the relationship. Yet many physicians and investigators of considerable renown still doubt the validity of the fat hypothesis, particularly relating the fat and cholesterol intake in the diet to the development of coronary heart disease. Some even question the relationship of blood cholesterol level to disease. (Certain studies have utilized only subjects in the older age category or have compared the quantity of atherosclerotic disease in a surgically removed vessel with serum measurements of cholesterol.) Most critics accept a relationship between the blood determination and the incidence of disease but doubt the relevance of dietary intake to blood cholesterol level. They have failed to consider both the factors that determine cholesterol level in populations living on relatively standardized diets and those that determine the differences between populations frequently living on distinctly different diets. More research is needed in both these fields, particularly to determine the factors that contribute to the individual cholesterol level.

Obesity and Atherosclerotic Disease

9

THE BELIEF THAT being overweight is hazardous to health is strongly ingrained in our society. It is supported by reasonably reliable statistics, first emphasized by life insurance company reports that highlighted the decreased life expectancy of persons who were relatively overweight (Marks, 1960). The additional cost of life insurance premiums of overweight persons has further impressed on everyone the risk of obesity. The maintenance of relatively low body weight is a necessity for those who wish to appear physically fit—and particularly in the case of women, for those who wish to be considered physically attractive.

Definitions of obesity suffer from the same difficulties as those relating to hypertension. Weight distribution is a continuous variable (Fig. 9-1). As observed in graphs of blood-pressure distribution, the normal curve is skewed to the right. There are more people who are overweight than underweight, since for the short term at least it is possible to put on considerable excess weight, whereas only a limited amount may be lost without serious consequences. Again, as with blood pressure, we may consider that the weight distribution curve includes a normal group—weight normally varying about a mean. This curve has then been altered by failure of a few individuals to gain weight, and by varying degrees of gain of many more. Thus weight gain

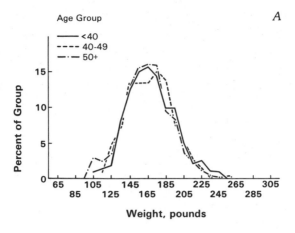

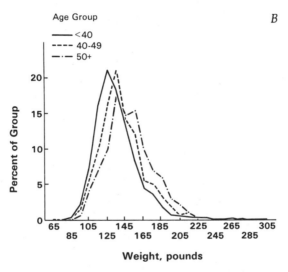

Fig. 9-1 *Distribution of weight of individuals in the Framingham Study. A, men; B, women.*

with age results in distribution curves that increase the skewing toward the higher values.

Body weight is a function of height and body build, sex, and degree of muscular development. However, the main factor is the degree of adiposity. If body fat could be removed, there would be little variability in weight in persons of the same height and body build. Presentation of the weight data to provide a meaningful estimate of adiposity has always posed problems (Mann, 1974). Simple crude weight measurements may give considerable information (especially if the values are exceptionally high or low), but the usual determinations do not provide as reliable an estimate of the degree of adiposity as desired. Elaborate techniques can be utilized to determine what percentage of the body mass is made up of fat, but these are impracticable for everyday medical application. Although skinfold thickness has been used as one method of measuring body fat, its value compared to function of weight is questionable. For these reasons derivations based on the crude weight (which provide a relative measure of the degree of obesity) have been most frequently utilized.

Since height, sex, and age are important factors in determining body weight, these characteristics can be used to assess "relative weight." Based on theoretical considerations in which the body may be viewed as a cylinder or a cone, some investigators have chosen to utilize other functions of height; the added value of such mathematical calculations is not obvious, however. If the weight of an individual is compared with a standard for the same age, sex, and height group to which he or she belongs, it is possible to calculate a relative weight that will relate the individual's weight to that of the group. Such standard weights have been compiled by insurance companies (the Metropolitan Life Weight Table, for instance) based on measurements obtained from their examiners. Others have been determined from specific groups of individuals—college students or other defined populations.

The set of values utilized in the Framingham Relative Weight Scale has been determined by comparing the weight of each individual to the *median* weight of all persons examined in the same age, sex, and height category. The degree to which an individual was above or below the median weight was then calculated. Thus, a Framingham subject who had a relative-weight value of 130 was 30 percent above the median weight of his or her same age, sex, and height group. A subject with a relative weight of 80 was 20 percent below the median weight for the group.

One difficulty with all such relative-weight scales is that the standard against which everyone is to be evaluated may be overweight or underweight, depending on the degree of overnutrition or undernutrition found in that population. Such relative-weight values thus characterize a subject in terms of others in the same group. Comparison with populations distinctly different in terms of their caloric nutritional state is not possible without reverting to the actual weight-for-height values. One criticism of the relative-weight scale used in Framingham is that this population was quite well nourished; any relative value is expressed in comparison to persons who would be overweight in a less affluent society.

The adverse effect of obesity may be brought about by several mechanisms, of which two are major. (1) Excess weight per se constitutes a physical burden to be carried about. Because of the effort required, the overweight person may become less active. If, however, the person performs a given task—going up a flight of stairs—he will perform *more* work than his thinner companion. If he does this work in the same time period, his energy output will be greater. (2) The stored body fat enters into the total metabolism. The body fat is not merely static, but is in the active pool of body nutrients where it is constantly being broken down and reformed. The fat must also be supplied with oxygen and nutrients, which increases the need for additional calories. Both of these factors undoubtedly contribute to some of the effects of excess weight.

Regardless of the mechanism by which adiposity contributes to disease and the question of what constitutes ideal weight, it is possible in a long-term epidemiologic study to determine how well subjects of different weight categories fare with respect to specific causes of morbidity and mortality. The subjects in the Framingham Study were weighed in a standard manner and classified according to their *relative* weight. Morbidity and mortality were then determined for differing categories of relative weight. With 24 years of follow-up it was possible to measure with considerable accuracy the effects excess weight might have on the various manifestations of atherosclerotic disease.

Relative Weight and Coronary Heart Disease

When all subjects developing any manifestations of coronary heart disease were grouped and compared with those not developing this disorder over a 24-year period, a clear-cut relationship of relative weight to the incidence of coronary heart disease was observed (Fig. 9-2). Male subjects who were 20 percent or more above the median weight were at about twice the risk of developing coronary heart disease as those below the median weight. In the "thin" category (below 80 relative weight) there was an even lower risk, indicating not only the advantage of avoiding obesity but of remaining distinctly below the expected weight. In women, at a much lower absolute risk, similar relative differences were noted in the incidence of coronary heart disease according to weight.

When an analysis was made reclassifying subjects by weight at each biennial examination, the findings were similar. Although the numbers of subjects in the high-relative-weight category were insufficient for adequate analysis, a comparison could be made in the weight categories below and above the median point, 100 (Fig. 9-3). In all age categories the incidence rate of coronary heart disease was 50 percent higher in subjects with greater relative weights.

Evaluation of the effects of weight on the development of the different clinical entities grouped under coronary heart disease revealed similarities to and differences from the total entity. This was to be expected, since excess weight acts both mechanically and metabolically.

Relative Weight and Angina Pectoris

Since the occurrence of angina pectoris is related to the immediate energy output, the obese person would be expected to demonstrate this symptom earlier in life than the nonobese. This would hold true even if the degree of atherosclerotic narrowing of the coronary artery were no greater, and the task undertaken were similar. After 24 years of observation the incidence rates of angina pectoris in both sexes were significantly higher the greater the relative weight of the subjects involved (Fig. 9-4). In addition, for both men and women, except in the youngest group, the average age of onset of symptoms was lower the greater the relative weight. In women who were 50-59 years old at the start of the study, the average age at which angina pectoris developed was four years earlier in those who were 20 percent above the median weight compared with those below the median weight. In men, even though the age differences were not as striking, the trend was in the same direction.

Relative Weight and Myocardial Infarction

In earlier reports from Framingham myocardial infarction did not appear to be importantly related to weight (Kannel et al., 1967). However, after 24 years of follow-up, an association became apparent (Fig. 9-5). In men in the older age groups the trend was reasonably consistent; no relationship was demonstrated in the 30-39 year group. In women a definite trend was seen in all age cohorts. Data on the average annual incidence rates, which correct for changes in weight at each examination, showed an even more consistent relation between relative weight and the incidence of myocardial infarction in both sexes (Fig. 9-6). In women the differences are less, possibly because of a greater degree of weight control, which would have the effect of placing subjects formerly overweight into lower weight categories.

The conclusion of a minimal effect of obesity on the development of myocardial infarction drawn earlier in the study was not justified by the results of 24 years of follow-up. Myocardial infarction is importantly related to body weight.

Relative Weight and Sudden Death

Earlier reports from Framingham showed a strong relation between excess weight and sudden death (Kannel et al., 1967), which is reiterated by analysis of the 24-year follow-up (Fig. 9-7). In men there was a steep gradient of risk with increasing relative weight. Those above the median weight had two to four times the risk of sudden death compared with those below that weight. In women, sudden death was too infrequent to permit this evaluation.

When analysis took into account changes in weight with time, a somewhat different picture emerged (Fig. 9-8). Much of the effect of excess weight appeared to be lost. An explanation for the discrepancy between the two methods of analysis may lie in the reclassification of subjects at each examination. A review of the weight status of subjects experiencing sudden death showed that a high percentage of these individuals had lost considerable weight in the two-year period prior to the event. Although there was no history of clinical symptoms, the loss of weight at this particular time suggests that these individuals may have experienced anginal discomfort, which prompted the weight loss.

Relative Weight and Cerebral Vascular Accidents

When the incidence of strokes of all types was analyzed in terms of relative weight, excess weight again appeared as an important factor. In both men and women observed over a 24-year period, the incidence rate of strokes of all types was greater the higher the relative weight. This same trend was observed when the analysis was confined to atherothrombotic brain infarction. Subjects 20 percent or more above the median relative weight had rates two to three times those of subjects below that weight (Fig. 9-9). When the analysis considered the change in weight status over the years, the excess risk in the overweight subjects still appeared. Comparison of those above and below median weight indicated about a 30 percent average annual excess rate of atherothrombotic brain infarction in the heavier male subjects at all ages. In women excess weight more than doubled the risk (Fig. 9-10).

(*continued on page 154*)

OBESITY AND ATHEROSCLEROTIC DISEASE

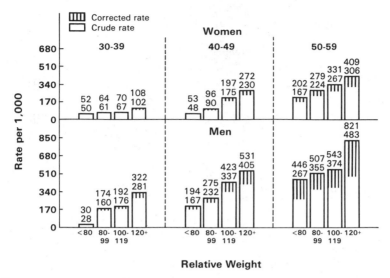

Fig. 9-2 *24-year incidence of coronary heart disease, by relative weight.*

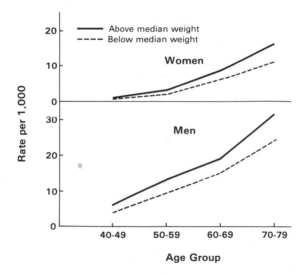

Fig. 9-3 *Average annual incidence of coronary heart disease, by weight category.*

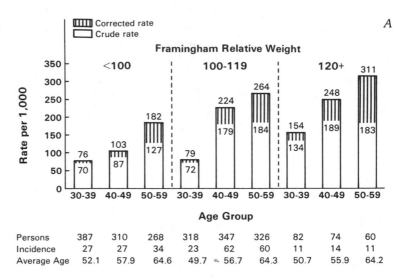

Persons	387	310	268	318	347	326	82	74	60
Incidence	27	27	34	23	62	60	11	14	11
Average Age	52.1	57.9	64.6	49.7	56.7	64.3	50.7	55.9	64.2

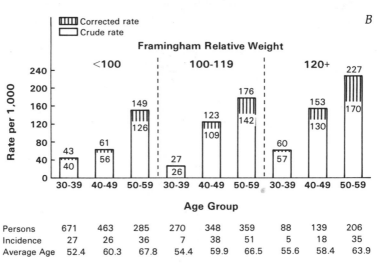

Persons	671	463	285	270	348	359	88	139	206
Incidence	27	26	36	7	38	51	5	18	35
Average Age	52.4	60.3	67.8	54.4	59.9	66.5	55.6	58.4	63.9

Fig. 9-4 *24-year incidence of angina pectoris, by relative weight of individuals age 30-59 at entry. A, men; B, women.*

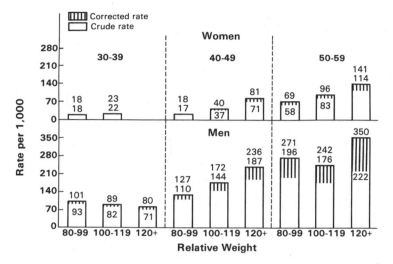

Fig. 9-5 *24-year incidence of myocardial infarction, by relative weight.*

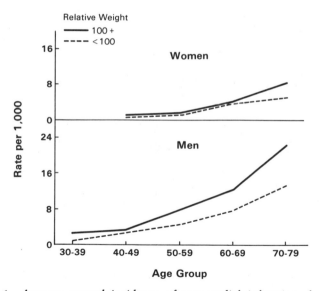

Fig. 9-6 *Average annual incidence of myocardial infarction, by relative weight category.*

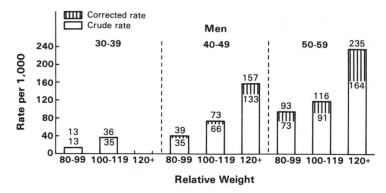

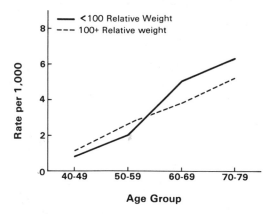

Fig. 9-7 *24-year incidence of sudden death, by relative weight, of men age 30-59 at entry.*

Fig. 9-8 *Average annual incidence of sudden death of men, by relative weight category.*

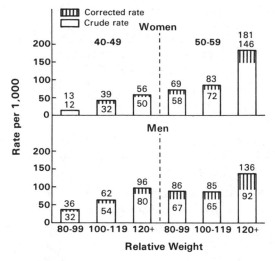

Fig. 9-9 *24-year incidence of atherothrombotic brain infarction, by relative weight.*

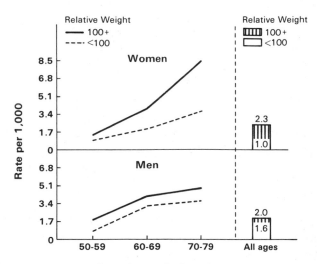

Fig. 9-10 *Average annual incidence of atherothrombotic brain infarction, by relative weight.*

Relative Weight and Peripheral Arterial Disease

Although in the younger men some association between weight and the development of intermittent claudication was apparent, the effect was not evident in the two older decades. In women no relationship showed up. When the average annual incidence at different ages was analyzed, no evidence of a deleterious effect of excess weight on the incidence of intermittent claudication was observed. One reason for this nonrelationship of peripheral arterial disease to weight may lie in the walking habits of the overweight. Tending to walk less and at a slower pace, they may not demonstrate any symptoms of claudication even if peripheral arterial disease is present. For whatever reason, excess weight did not contribute importantly to the incidence of intermittent claudication. However, for the other manifestations of atherosclerotic disease excess weight played an important role.

Relative Weight and Other Risk Factors

The effect of obesity may be related to other risk factors such as blood pressure and blood lipids. Before it is concluded that the hazards of obesity result from excess weight in itself, the relationship between weight and the various other risk factors needs to be analyzed. The values for blood pressure, serum cholesterol, physical activity index, and uric acid in the several weight categories are presented in Table 9-1. Data on cigarette consumption are not included because no significant differences were found.

RELATIVE WEIGHT AND BLOOD PRESSURE

The importance of body weight, the only variable that had a major effect on blood-pressure level, has been discussed previously. Very clearly in each age decade, and for both men and women, body weight was firmly related to systolic and diastolic blood-pressure level. The weight-related differences were not only statistically significant but were of sufficient magnitude to suggest that this relationship could explain some of the risk associated with adiposity. The magnitude of the weight-blood-pressure relationship indicated that any attempt to lower blood pressure should involve weight reduction as a primary effort.

OBESITY AND ATHEROSCLEROTIC DISEASE

Table 9-1 Risk factors in the population according to relative weight.

Relative weight[a]	Blood pressure		Cholesterol (mg %)	Physical activity index[b]	Uric acid (mg %)
	Systolic (mm Hg)	Diastolic (mm Hg)			
			MEN		
			AGE 30-39		
< 100	128	80	208	35	4.6
100-129	135	87	226	34	5.1
130+	145	94	226	34	6.1
			AGE 40-49		
< 100	132	83	222	34	4.6
100-129	140	90	230	33	5.1
130+	153	96	232	38	7.0
			AGE 50-59		
< 100	138	85	223	33	4.4
100-129	146	90	230	32	5.1
130+	163	100	219	31	5.5
			WOMEN		
			AGE 30-39		
< 100	122	79	202	32	3.4
100-129	126	81	208	32	3.7
130+	142	90	204	31	4.4
			AGE 40-49		
< 100	130	81	222	31	3.6
100-129	140	88	231	31	3.8
130+	156	95	237	31	4.2
			AGE 50-59		
< 100	146	88	252	30	3.7
100-129	152	90	253	30	4.2
130+	171	100	241	29	4.5

[a]Weight compared to the median weight for the appropriate sex and height group.
[b]Derived from the history of usual 24-hour activity (see Chapter 10 for details).

Relative Weight and Serum Cholesterol

The relation between body weight and serum cholesterol level was much weaker than in the case of blood pressure. In the youngest decade of men below the median weight, the serum cholesterol levels were not only significantly lower (208 mg%) than the mean values for that age group (223 mg%), but the difference was sufficiently great that in this age group of men it could have contributed to the effect of weight on disease development. The differences observed in other decades in both men and women, though significant, were of far smaller magnitude.

Relative Weight and Other Factors

Differences in physical activity were slight and much smaller than might be expected in view of the assumed sedentary behavior of many obese persons. That excess weight is a factor in the total metabolism is attested to by the difference in average uric acid values found in the several weight categories. In every age group and in both sexes the uric acid values increased with increasing weight. Clearly, the major factor associated with weight is blood pressure, with a weaker relation to cholesterol, physical activity, and uric acid level. Even if these factors are taken into consideration, however, there remains an effect of excess weight that must be attributed to the adiposity itself.

One aspect of obesity that has not received sufficient attention is the manner in which the excess weight is acquired. Weight is added by caloric intake above that which is needed. The calories can come from carbohydrate, protein, fat, or any combination of these. The fat can be of relative degrees of saturation. Although it can be assumed that most obese persons eat to excess in all categories of dietary intake, it is conceivable that the person whose obesity resulted from a high fat intake, especially from saturated animal fat, might be affecting his metabolic state more adversely than the individual whose adiposity was largely caused by carbohydrate intake or relatively unsaturated fat. Measurements of the chemical structure of body fat provide useful information if the dietary intake has been sufficiently varied to produce differences in the fat composition. Unfortunately we have no data from the Framingham Study that bear directly on this question.

Physical Activity and
Cardiovascular Disease

10

AMONG THE SEVERAL HYPOTHESES that have been proposed linking way of life to the development of cardiovascular disease, one of the most popular has involved physical activity. People have always judged work to be a virtue and laziness a vice. Physical educators believe that muscular exertion is beneficial to the total metabolism. Their concepts are based largely on what they would like to believe, rather than on careful evaluation of any benefits. Calisthenics and sports, together with other athletic training, may be of recreational value, but the alleged positive effect of such activities on health is probably greatly exaggerated. Performance of hard physical work or any high-energy exercise for limited periods of time may be helpful in conditioning the cardiovascular system to adjust efficiently to the short-term demands made on it. The result of such conditioning is an ability to perform work with a smaller rise in pulse rate, blood pressure, and respiratory rate.

The above type of physical activity should be distinguished from the steady performance of labor which, although calling for only small increments in cardiac work, does so for long periods of time. The total metabolic effect of such work over 24 hours, measured by calories burned, may be much greater than the effect of short bursts of high-energy-output exercise. The sedentary office worker who runs for 20 minutes a day may be able to respond much better to immediate exertion than a carpenter or coal miner, although the total energy output of the latter is markedly higher. Both types of physical activity have beneficial, but not necessarily similar, effects. The person who has conditioned his cardiovascular system to perform work with a smaller rise in pulse rate may expect to delay the onset of anginal symptoms even in the presence of coronary narrowing. An increased total 24-hour metabolism will modify the oxidation and storage of carbohydrate, fat, and protein. This may have an effect not only on such obvious factors as adiposity but on the atherosclerotic process itself. The desirability of physical work to improve total metabolism has been supported by evidence that persons with diabetes mellitus can control the disease better if they perform muscular work: their diet may be liberalized and less insulin needed.

Unfortunately, data supporting the belief in the health benefits of physical activity are difficult to obtain. Most of the programs promoted by physical educationists are pursued only by the young and are abandoned when they reach an age when major benefits might be realized. Some of those exposed to such physical training presumably continue to follow the program after leaving school or college. Studies of older men who engaged in various sports while in college suggest some benefit of regular exercise (Paffenbarger et al., 1966). One problem that makes assessment of such data extremely difficult is the self-selection involved. Only those who are particularly fitted to engage in sports or other athletic activities choose or are chosen to do so. Comparison of athletes with nonathletes may reflect a selection of the cohort more than the result of the exercise involved.

Physical exertion has a marked effect on the cardiovascular system. There is a rise in blood pressure, an increase in pulse rate, peripheral vasodilatation, increased cardiac output, and increased respiratory rate—all aimed at supplying oxygen to the working muscles. With training, a given task can be performed with a lesser cardiovascular response. One of the effects of exercise, both short term and long term, is the burning of additional calories with resultant weight loss.

Very early in the Framingham Study consideration was given to the desirability of assessing the physical energy output of the subjects. Very few people in our population were engaging in athletics or physical exercise as such. If differences were to be found, it would be in the total energy output. But there was reason to believe that even here marked differences might not be found. Nevertheless, a decision was made to assess this aspect of physical activity as the only one measurable, albeit crudely. This was undertaken at the fourth biennial examination.

Each subject was questioned regarding the number of hours spent in sleep and recumbent resting, sitting, standing, walking on the level, and at increasingly arduous tasks. From this the usual 24-hour energy output was determined by weighting the several levels of activity on the basis of the known oxygen consumption required. The lowest possible point on the scale was 24, which would indicate either sleep or recumbency for the entire day. Since remaining sedentary or walking on the level does not call for much excess oxygen consumption and most of the population was relatively inactive, many scores were not far above this minimal level.

Relation of Physical Activity to Other Risk Factors

Examination of the relationship between physical activity as determined in the Framingham population and other risk factors did not suggest any important association (Table 10-1). The most consistent relationship was with weight, in which there was a definite trend downward with increased physical activity in men in all age groups. In women the trend was similar except in subjects age 40-49. The blood-pressure trends were not consistent but favored a slightly lower systolic pressure in the more active. Overall there was no indication that whatever the relation of physical activity to disease outcome, it was being mediated through other risk factor associations. The lack of correlation, other than the slight effect on blood pressure and relative weight, was strengthened by the fact that the breaks used in the classification of the physical activity index were such as to produce only small numbers of subjects in the high and low categories. These represent the extremes of the distribution curve. Failure to demonstrate a more important relationship may be a result of the narrow range of values assigned to physical activity, which indicated very little difference in this characteristic from person to person, except for small numbers of men engag-

Table 10-1 Interrelationship of physical activity in men with other risk factors. (The physical activity index was not significantly related to cholesterol level, uric acid level, or smoking habits.)

Physical activity index	Blood pressure		Relative weight
	Systolic (mm Hg)	Diastolic (mm Hg)	
AGE 30-39			
<27	128	82	104
27-37	131	84	101
38+	133	84	100
AGE 40-49			
<27	140	88	106
27-37	136	87	102
38+	134	86	101
AGE 50-59			
<27	149	90	103
27-37	141	87	102
38+	143	87	101

ing in more strenuous exertion (Fig. 10-1). It might also reflect the difficulty of accurately measuring physical activity by the methodology used.

Physical Activity and Atherosclerotic Disease

Previous reports from Framingham have indicated a beneficial effect of higher levels of exertion as measured by the physical activity index. The benefits first observed were related primarily to survival after the development of myocardial infarction rather than to a diminished incidence of the disease (Dawber, 1973). Because of the relatively narrow range of index figures, separation of the population into distinctly different groups with regard to this factor was difficult. The classification we have used attempts to separate the minimally active from the maximally active, with a large group ("usually active") in between having limited variability in activity indexes.

Physical Activity and Coronary Heart Disease

In men the sedentary individuals had approximately three times the rate of coronary heart disease observed in the most active (Fig. 10-2). In women a relationship was also found with a ratio of over 2.5 to one. The age of onset generally was younger in the least active individuals, which further accentuated the difference in incidence rates.

When the analysis was made in terms of average annual incidence, there was a clear gradient of risk for both men and women at all the ages in which incidence was sufficient for evaluation (Fig. 10-3). The least active group had two to three times the incidence of coronary heart disease compared to the most active. Lesser differences were found between usually active and the most vigorous. Since almost all attempts to increase activity would advance an individual from the usual group to the most active, these data suggest limited benefits from the added level of exercise. They do, however, indicate a distinct advantage of being other than strictly sedentary.

Physical Activity and Myocardial Infarction

The 24-year incidence rates of myocardial infarction showed a relation to physical activity similar to that seen for all coronary heart disease (Fig. 10-4). The highest rates were found in the small sedentary group. Differences in age of onset were not consistent. Again, the differences observed between the usually active and the most active were minimal.

Average annual incidence rates in men followed the pattern observed for all coronary heart disease, with little difference between the usually active and more active individuals but with a considerable excess incidence in the sedentary group (Fig. 10-5). This analysis excluded subjects with angina pectoris who, if included, might have confused the evaluation, since more of them would probably have fallen into the sedentary group.

Physical Activity and Angina Pectoris

Although on theoretical grounds angina pectoris should be most closely related to physical activity in men, the gradient with increasing activity was similar to all coronary heart disease (Fig. 10-6). In women no significant relationship was noted.

Even in men the difference in incidence between the most active and the usually active subjects was minimal. Interpretation of these data was difficult, since a number of subjects may have deliberately decreased their physical activity to avoid anginal symptoms and underreported their usual activity.

The average annual incidence rates in men for all ages showed a distinctly higher figure in the least active group (Fig. 10-7). In women the numbers were too small for analysis except in the 50-59 decade, where a gradient of risk was also observed.

Physical Activity and Sudden Death

Too few subjects developed sudden death in the high and low physical-activity categories to estimate reliable rates. There was a suggestion that the sudden death rate was low in the most active men. The average annual rate could be calculated only for the entire period, but did show a decreased gradient of risk from more active to sedentary.

Physical Activity and Peripheral Arterial Disease

No evidence of a relationship between physical activity status and intermittent claudication was found. The analysis was confounded by the obvious fact that people developing any manifestations of leg discomfort would tend to remain inactive.

Physical Activity and Atherothrombotic Brain Infarction

The limited numbers of subjects developing atherothrombotic brain infarction in the younger age categories precluded analysis below the age 50-59 cohort (Fig. 10-8). In that age group, followed for 24 years, there was a gradient of risk favoring the most physically active men. Average annual incidence for the entire period of the study showed a higher rate of atherothrombotic brain infarction in the sedentary subjects.

(continued on page 171)

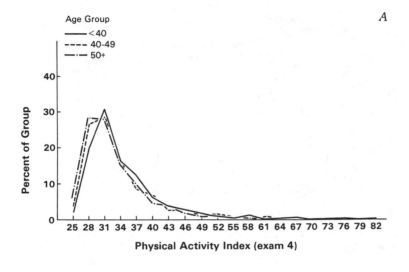

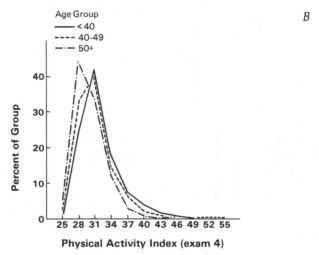

Fig. 10-1 *Distribution of physical activity index. A, men; B, women.*

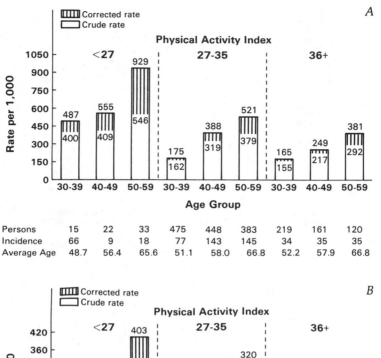

Persons	15	22	33	475	448	383	219	161	120
Incidence	66	9	18	77	143	145	34	35	35
Average Age	48.7	56.4	65.6	51.1	58.0	66.8	52.2	57.9	66.8

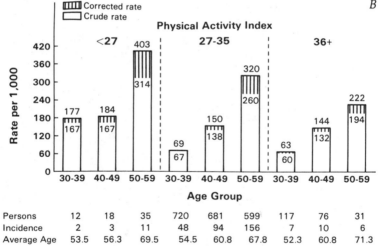

Persons	12	18	35	720	681	599	117	76	31
Incidence	2	3	11	48	94	156	7	10	6
Average Age	53.5	56.3	69.5	54.5	60.8	67.8	52.3	60.8	71.3

Fig. 10-2 *24-year incidence of coronary heart disease, by physical activity index of individuals age 30-59 at entry. A, men; B, women.*

PHYSICAL ACTIVITY AND CARDIOVASCULAR DISEASE

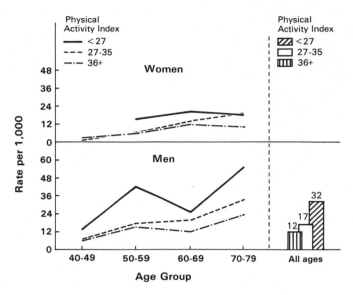

Fig. 10-3 *Average annual incidence of coronary heart disease, by physical activity index.*

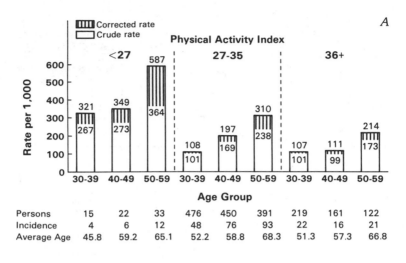

Persons	15	22	33	476	450	391	219	161	122
Incidence	4	6	12	48	76	93	22	16	21
Average Age	45.8	59.2	65.1	52.2	58.8	68.3	51.3	57.3	66.8

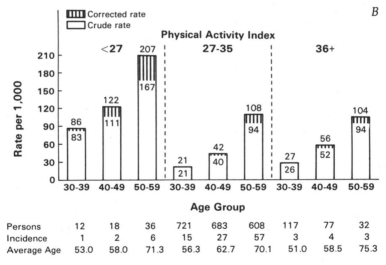

Persons	12	18	36	721	683	608	117	77	32
Incidence	1	2	6	15	27	57	3	4	3
Average Age	53.0	58.0	71.3	56.3	62.7	70.1	51.0	58.5	75.3

Fig. 10-4 *24-year incidence of myocardial infarction, by physical activity index of individuals age 30-59 at entry. A, men; B, women.*

PHYSICAL ACTIVITY AND CARDIOVASCULAR DISEASE

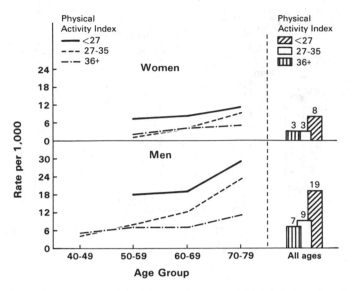

Fig. 10-5 *Average annual incidence of myocardial infarction, by physical activity index.*

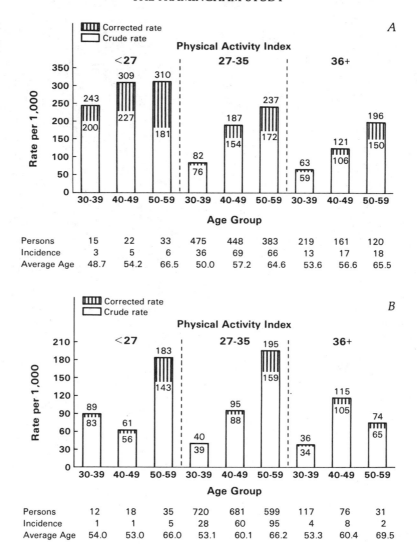

Fig. 10-6 *24-year incidence of angina pectoris, by physical activity index of individuals age 30-59 at entry. A, men; B, women.*

PHYSICAL ACTIVITY AND CARDIOVASCULAR DISEASE

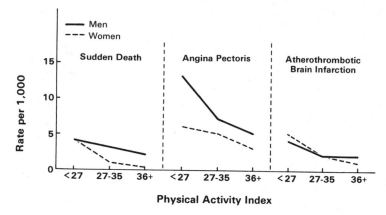

Fig. 10-7 *Average annual incidence of manifestations of cardiovascular disease, by physical activity index.*

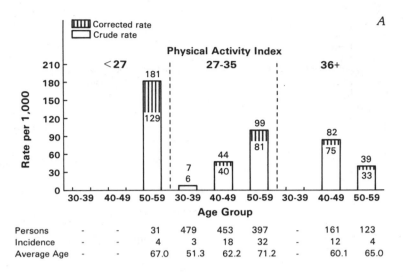

Persons	-	-	31	479	453	397	-	161	123
Incidence	-	-	4	3	18	32	-	12	4
Average Age	-	-	67.0	51.3	62.2	71.2	-	60.1	65.0

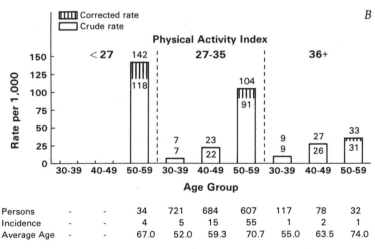

Persons	-	-	34	721	684	607	117	78	32
Incidence	-	-	4	5	15	55	1	2	1
Average Age	-	-	67.0	52.0	59.3	70.7	55.0	63.5	74.0

Fig. 10-8 *24-year incidence of atherothrombotic brain infarction, by physical activity index of individuals age 30-59 at entry. A, men; B, women.*

Summary

The data suggested distinct benefit from avoiding the sedentary life. The value of increasing activity above moderate involvement was less apparent; the decreased risk in the most active group was modest. However, there were very few individuals in the entire Framingham population who engaged in extremely strenuous work or high levels of physical exercise. These data therefore cannot corroborate the wisdom of undertaking the programs of high-energy-output exercise now being encouraged. Prospective studies of such programs are needed to determine their benefit both qualitatively and quantitatively.

Tobacco and Cardiovascular Disease

11

AT THE TIME the Framingham Study was being planned, there was no hard evidence that the use of tobacco was responsible for any long-term damage to the cardiovascular system. The acute effects of smoking on the heart and blood vessels had been clearly demonstrated by numerous studies (Dawber, 1960). These effects consisted primarily in a rise in pulse rate, a slight elevation of blood pressure, and some increase in cardiac output—all changes associated with peripheral arteriolar constriction. Premature beats were also frequently observed. Such effects were more pronounced in people who smoked cigarettes than in those who smoked pipes or cigars. There was reason to believe that any factor which produced acute changes might with repeated exposure adversely affect the cardiovascular system over the long term. Some of the acute effects of smoking, particularly of cigarettes, could also be produced by the injection of equivalent amounts of nicotine. As an adrenergic drug, it could well be considered responsible for the immediate cardiovascular effects of tobacco smoking.

In 1950 the fact that pipe, cigar, and cigarette smoke differed considerably in the quality and quantity of the physical and chemical constituents of the smoke was not fully appreciated. Nor were the considerable variations in the inhalation practices of pipe, cigar, and cigarette smokers recognized. However, because of possible differences on this basis, it appeared desirable to collect data by type of smoking. Information obtained at several examinations has permitted classification into nonsmokers; ex-smokers; and cigarette, pipe, and cigar smokers. The amount of smoking (number of cigarettes, pipes, cigars per day) was also quantified. The smoking habits of the population have changed during the 24 years, with a significant drop in the percentage of cigarette smokers in the male population (Gordon et al., 1975).

A breakdown of the Framingham population according to smoking practices showed the predominance of cigarette smoking in the male population, with considerably less tobacco usage by the women, especially in the older age groups. Because of the widespread usage of tobacco in this population the number of nonsmokers was relatively small. A long period of observation was needed to accumulate sufficient data to test a possible effect of smoking on coronary heart disease. In fact, the first publications required the combination of two studies—ours and one in Albany, New York—to provide sufficient numbers of subjects with disease in the various subgroups (Doyle et al., 1962, 1964).

With the passage of time and the opportunity to observe disease development over a longer period, considerable data have been collected that clearly implicate tobacco usage in atherosclerotic disease. Observations in the later years of the study, when many of the subjects had become elderly, indicated limitations of the adverse effect of smoking. There were valid reasons to separate the subcategories of smoking, at least in terms of nonsmokers, cigarette smokers, and cigar and pipe smokers. Quantitation of the amount of smoking in the several categories also appeared advisable. In retrospect, the inhalation practices of the smokers should have been determined. The assumption that all smokers inhale was of course incorrect, since pipe and cigar smokers rarely do so while almost all cigarette smokers who smoke a pack or more per day inhale. The degree of inhalation can readily be measured by determining the carbon monoxide content of the blood after exposure to smoke. Although this test is a simple one performed in the doctor's office, it was not available in 1950. It has enabled us to determine that cigarette smokers evidence approximately 30 parts per million of carbon monoxide in their blood, whereas pipe and cigar smokers have practically none. An exception occurred in those cigar or pipe smokers who were former cigarette smokers and whose carbon monoxide content was approximately 5 parts per million. Those who combine smoking practices, including cigarettes, may also be expected to demonstrate carbon monoxide in the blood.

Tobacco Smoking and Coronary Heart Disease

The first analysis of tobacco smoking showed rather clearly that the adverse effects of smoking on coronary heart disease development appeared only in those individuals who smoked cigarettes (Doyle et al., 1964). In such individuals it was found that there was a higher rate of coronary heart disease particularly attributable to myocardial infarction and sudden death. The correlation of cigarette smoking and angina pectoris was relatively slight. Subsequent analyses have pretty much confirmed the previous findings, but have shown a stronger relationship between cigarette smoking and angina pectoris; they have also indicated a diminishing effect on all types of coronary heart disease with age (Gordon et al., 1974).

After 24 years of observation we are now able to assess the long-term effect of tobacco smoking on coronary heart disease and to indicate the magnitude of this effect in the several age groups studied. Previous comparison of the incidence rates of coronary heart disease in the various smoking categories demonstrated no relation of pipe smoking or cigar smoking to coronary heart disease. This was consistent with the noninhalation practices of such smokers rather than any benign character of the smoke from these two forms of tobacco. (In fact, such smoke contains higher percentages of carbon monoxide and nicotine.) The increased rate of coronary heart disease was found only in those who smoked cigarettes.

A reanalysis of cigarette smoking practices showed a strong relationship of the smoking habit to coronary heart disease, although a diminishing effect with age (Fig. 11-1). The younger male cigarette smokers had twice the rate of the nonsmokers. In the group age 40-49 years the relationship was weaker, and in the oldest age group no association was seen. Among women no significant effect of smoking was observed. The diminishing effect with age in men naturally decreases the difference between the incidence rates in smokers and in nonsmokers the longer the follow-up period. Another factor of importance is the age of onset of coronary heart disease, which is earlier in cigarette smokers by approximately two and one-half years (Table 11-1). Among women no significant effect of smoking was observed.

The above data, based on smoking habits at initial examination, assumed continuation of these habits over the period of observation. Whereas very few nonsmokers take up smoking after reaching the age of subjects in this study, there has been an increasing number of men who have changed their smoking habits or given up smoking altogether. If the analysis is made to determine the risk in narrower age brackets and the smoking status is based on practices much closer in time to the event, a similar although more potent effect of cigarette smoking is observed (Fig. 11-2). The average annual rate of coronary heart disease development in male cigarette smokers was approximately three times that of nonsmokers in both the 30-39 and 40-49 age groups. It was about twice the rate in the 50-59 age group and decreased further with age. The average annual rates for all ages, while still somewhat higher for cigarette smokers (11.9), was not greatly different than for nonsmokers (10.1). This is of course because although the *relative risk* of cigarette smokers is much higher than that of nonsmokers, the effect is most noticeable in the younger subjects where the *absolute risk* is low.

Among male cigarette smokers there was also a trend upward in risk of coronary heart disease with increased cigarette smoking (Fig. 11-3). This was clearly demonstrated in the youngest

Table 11-1 Average age of onset of coronary heart disease (other than angina pectoris) in male smokers and nonsmokers of cigarettes.

Smoke cigarettes	Age cohort		
	30-39	40-49	50-59
Yes	50.1	56.7	67.0
No	52.8	60.3	65.3

decade of smokers, but the gradient had largely disappeared by age 60. The gradient of risk was most pronounced in comparing nonsmokers with those who smoked one or more packs per day (20 or more cigarettes); in the younger men the risk was about four times greater than in nonsmokers.

CIGARETTE SMOKING AND RISK OF MYOCARDIAL INFARCTION

Since the effect of cigarette smoking may differ in the various clinical entities that make up the coronary heart disease category, the relationship in each of these disorders should be examined separately. Among men the major entity contributing to this category was myocardial infarction. Its relation to cigarette smoking at initial examination is indicated in Fig. 11-4. Cigarette smoking was clearly a risk factor for the development of myocardial infarction in men age 30-39 observed over a 24-year period (until these men reached 54-63), with the risk in cigarette smokers approximately three times that in non-cigarette smokers. Among men in the decade 40-49 at the time of entry into the study, the risk in cigarette smokers was approximately twice that in nonsmokers. Above the age of 50 no significant difference was noted, although the trend appeared to be reversing itself with a higher rate in the nonsmokers. Again, the age of onset of myocardial infarction was earlier in the smokers (56.4 years versus 63.2 in the 40-49 age cohort). Among women— who have a much lower absolute risk of myocardial infarction —no significant differences were noted between smokers and nonsmokers.

Thus cigarette smoking was an important factor in the development of myocardial infarction in men below age 50 observed over a 24-year period. Above that age it lost its importance. Because half of the myocardial infarction occurred in older men, the overall rate in all ages was not greatly different for smokers than for nonsmokers. Any discussion of the importance of cigarette smoking in the development of myocardial infarction must consider the age group involved.

When the analysis utilized an average annual incidence for shorter periods of time, the importance of the relationship in the younger subjects again was well demonstrated (Fig. 11-5). This analysis involving ten-year intervals took into consideration changes in smoking habits. Cigarette smoking was an important factor up to the age of 60, with a difference of as much as four to one in the younger age groups. As before, the overall effect was diminished by the high absolute incidence rates in the older age groups in which the risk of cigarette smoking was minimal.

When the quantity of cigarettes smoked was examined, there was a clear-cut gradient in men 40-49 years old from non-cigarette smokers to those who smoked a pack or more daily (Fig. 11-6). This gradient was less steep in the 50-59 year old men and was lost altogether above age 60.

As might be expected, no relation of myocardial infarction to cigar or pipe smoking was observed.

CIGARETTE SMOKING AND SUDDEN DEATH

Of all the manifestations of coronary heart disease after 24 years of follow-up, sudden death has been found most strongly related to cigarette smoking. Among cigarette smokers the rate of sudden death in the youngest decade was almost four times greater than that of nonsmokers (Fig. 11-7). The rate was about twice as high in the older age groups, a relationship that held true for the entire population. Earlier onset of sudden death in the smokers was also observed (Table 11-2). In women no relationship was apparent.

When the quantity of cigarettes smoked was taken into consideration, there was also a gradient of risk with increased cigarette consumption in the youngest decade; in the older subjects the gradient was not apparent. When the analysis utilized shorter periods of follow-up and took into consideration changes in smoking habits, the importance of the effect of cigarette smoking on sudden death became even more evident. At any age the sudden death rate was greater in cigarette smokers

Table 11-2 Cigarette smoking and average age of onset of sudden death in men.

Smoke cigarettes	Age cohort		
	30-39	40-49	50-59
Yes	50.1	57.5	65.5
No	51.0	60.8	68.8

by about two to one. This held even for the older subjects (70-79 age group), although the number involved was small.

Two major differences in the effect of cigarette smoking on sudden death compared to other manifestations of coronary heart disease stand out. The relationship is stronger, and although diminished it is not lost with age. The increased ischemia of the myocardium produced by the higher carbon monoxide content of the blood and the increased myocardial irritability from nicotine are possible contributory mechanisms. The data certainly suggest that the effect of cigarette smoking on sudden death does not result from differences in coronary atherosclerosis but rather from a direct effect on the myocardium itself. This, in turn, suggests that the risk of sudden death may be decreased by quitting smoking regardless of age.

CIGARETTE SMOKING AND ANGINA PECTORIS

In the early reports from the Framingham Study the effect of cigarette smoking on the incidence of angina pectoris appeared to be relatively slight. As time went by, it became increasingly clear that although the effect of cigarette smoking was weaker than in some other manifestations of coronary heart disease, there was nevertheless a definite relationship, particularly in the younger subjects (Fig. 11-8). In the youngest decade the risk in cigarette smokers of developing angina pectoris was about twice that in nonsmokers, with a smaller difference in the older age groups. Similarly, a gradient of risk was observed from the nonsmokers to those who smoked over a pack a day in both the 30-39 and 40-49 age cohorts. Once again, no effects showed up in women.

Smoking and Stroke

The effect of tobacco smoking on the development of stroke and its various underlying entities was relatively small. When all cerebral vascular accidents (excluding transient ischemic attacks) were analyzed in terms of tobacco smoking, there was only a very slight excess incidence in cigarette smokers (Fig. 11-9). Although there was always a higher rate in smokers, the differences were not significant. The small numbers of cigar and pipe smokers developing stroke made analysis of this type of tobacco use difficult; still there appeared to be no reason to implicate cigar or pipe smoking.

When we utilized shorter periods of follow-up and took into account changes in smoking habits, we again observed a slightly higher rate of stroke in the cigarette smokers, but this was neither statistically significant nor clinically important. And in terms of the number of cigarettes smoked, no consistent gradient was apparent.

SMOKING AND ATHEROSCLEROTIC BRAIN INFARCTION

When the thrombotic stroke group alone was analyzed, the relationship was similar to that found in the total cerebral vascular accident group. The incidence of atherothrombotic brain infarction in cigarette smokers was slightly but consistently above that found in nonsmokers in all age groups, based on smoking habits at initial examination. No regular gradient was observed when the number of cigarettes smoked was taken into account. On shorter term follow-up, with the changes in smoking habits taken into consideration, a slight increase in average annual incidence of atherothrombotic brain infarction was also apparent in the cigarette smokers, but the increased risk was of such limited magnitude that no clinical importance should be attached. Similarly, little evidence emerged of any relationship to the number of cigarettes smoked. Thus, it was apparent that the role of tobacco smoking in general, and cigarette smoking in particular, in the development of stroke and atherothrombotic brain infarction is minor. Possible reasons for this will be considered below.

Smoking and Peripheral Arterial Disease

The importance of tobacco smoking to the development and progression of peripheral arterial disease has long been recognized. This relationship gave rise to the concept that arterial disease of the lower extremities was in many ways distinct from the usual atherosclerotic process elsewhere in the body. The possibility that peripheral arteriolar vasospasm was the result of sensitivity to nicotine and other ingredients in tobacco smoke was considered.

An opportunity to observe the effect of tobacco smoking in the development of peripheral arterial disease was provided in the Framingham Study and is one of the reasons for the attempts to continue the study over as long a time as possible. As indicated previously, the manifestation of peripheral arterial disease utilized in the Framingham analyses has been intermittent claudication. Based on 24 years of observation and in terms of smoking habits at initial examination, the incidence rates of this manifestation in male cigarette smokers were over twice that observed in nonsmokers. In the older age groups, in which the disease was most common, the rate was about three to one (Fig. 11-10). No relationship was noted in women. Although the number of subjects involved was small, there appeared to be a possible increased risk of intermittent claudication in cigar but not in pipe smokers. No gradient of risk was observed in the cigarette smokers according to amount smoked.

When the analysis was based on shorter term follow-up, and changes in smoking habits taken into account, a similar picture was seen. The average annual rate in the 50-69 year old male cigarette smokers was approximately twice that in the non-cigarette smokers (Fig. 11-11). Even among older women (60-79) the rate of development of intermittent claudication in cigarette smokers was twice that in nonsmokers. No consistent gradient among cigarette smokers was observed, although higher rates were noted in those smoking more than a pack of cigarettes per day.

Peripheral arterial disease is therefore clearly related to the cigarette smoking habit in all age groups of men. In women, in whom cigarette smoking had not been an important factor in the development of other manifestations of atherosclerotic disease, there appeared to be a relationship to intermittent claudication.

(*continued on page 186*)

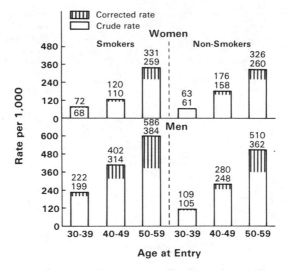

Fig. 11-1 *24-year incidence of coronary heart disease, by cigarette smoking status.*

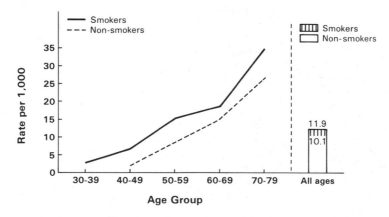

Fig. 11-2 *Average annual incidence of coronary heart disease in men, by cigarette smoking status.*

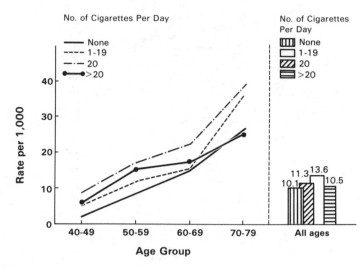

Fig. 11-3 *Average annual incidence of coronary heart disease in men, by amount of smoking.*

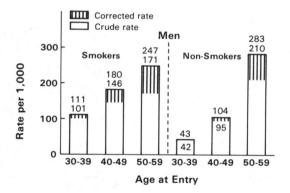

Fig. 11-4 *24-year incidence of myocardial infarction in men, by cigarette smoking status.*

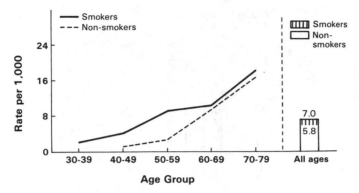

Fig. 11-5 *Average annual incidence of myocardial infarction in men, by cigarette smoking status.*

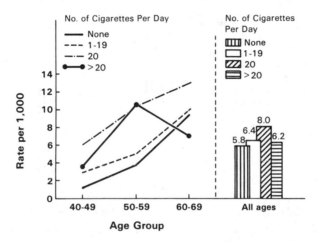

Fig. 11-6 *Average annual incidence of myocardial infarction in men, by amount of smoking.*

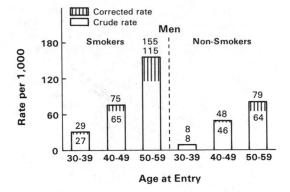

Fig. 11-7   *24-year incidence of sudden death in men, by cigarette smoking status.*

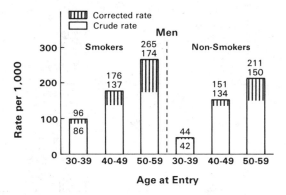

Fig. 11-8   *24-year incidence of angina pectoris in men, by cigarette smoking status.*

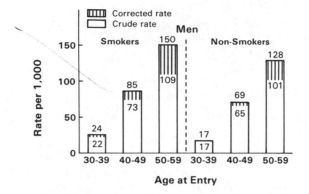

Fig. 11-9   *24-year incidence of cerebral vascular accident in men, by cigarette smoking status.*

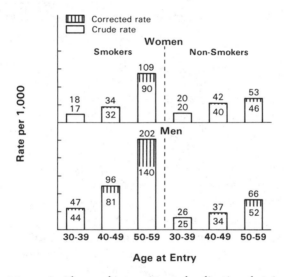

Fig. 11-10   *24-year incidence of intermittent claudication, by cigarette smoking status.*

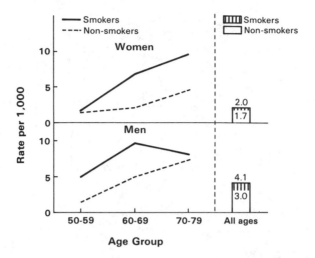

Fig. 11-11 *Average annual incidence of intermittent claudication, by ciga-rette smoking status.*

Summary and Discussion

The relation of tobacco usage to cardiovascular disease development has been somewhat clarified by long-term studies such as the one conducted in Framingham. *Cigarette* smoking stands out as the habit that is hazardous in men. The development of all types of coronary heart disease was higher in male cigarette smokers than in nonsmokers, but the difference decreased with age until it became nil in the older subjects (over 65 years). The major clinical entities involved are myocardial infarction and sudden death, in which the incidence rate in smokers compared to nonsmokers was the highest. In stroke and atherothrombotic brain infarction only a slight difference was noted between cigarette smokers and nonsmokers. In peripheral arterial disease a strong relationship favoring the non-cigarette smokers was apparent. Neither pipe nor cigar smoking was related to cardiovascular disease incidence.

The reasons for the relation of tobacco usage to cardiovascular disease are still not completely understood. However, certain new knowledge of differences among the various categories of smokers throws some light on the subject. At the start of the study our inclination was to group all users of tobacco together; then it became clear that there were important differences in the smoke content of different forms of tobacco. Most important, however, were variations in the inhalation practices of the smokers. Unfortunately we did not inquire regarding these practices early in the study. Since then, however, it has been adequately demonstrated that, as a group, cigar and pipe smokers do not inhale the smoke (Dawber, 1976). Some absorption of nicotine does occur in the mouth, but it is minimal. As demonstrated by carbon monoxide levels in the blood, neither cigar nor pipe smokers absorb any of this noxious gas (although the carbon monoxide content of cigar and pipe smoke is higher than that of cigarettes). Interestingly, among cigar and pipe smokers who take up this form of tobacco use *after* quitting cigarettes, there are measurable amounts of carbon monoxide in the blood —which indicates some inhalation by this particular group of smokers.

Among cigarette smokers the number used is not distributed normally; approximately 75 percent of the men reported smoking 20 or more cigarettes per day (33 percent over a pack per day). At that rate it is possible to demonstrate, on the basis of carbon monoxide blood levels, that inhalation has almost always taken place. Among women, however, the percentage who smoked one or more packs of cigarettes per day was only about 35, with only 8 percent admitting to more than a pack per day. Of the 65 percent of women who smoked less than 20 cigarettes a day, many smoked only two or three. Thus it is reasonable to conclude that among the women cigarette smokers in this population, only a small percentage inhaled. The combination of this knowledge and the Framingham data make it apparent that the inhalation of tobacco smoke—which in effect means cigarette smoke—is the hazardous practice so far as cardiovascular disease is concerned.

Numerous chemicals have been identified in tobacco smoke, some of which may be responsible for the development of lung cancer and other pulmonary diseases. Others may be implicated in the development of cardiovascular diseases. Interest has focused primarily on nicotine and carbon monoxide, which are absorbed into the blood stream from tobacco smoke inhaled into the lungs. Both of these agents are toxic and produce known effects. Carbon monoxide, by combining with hemoglobin and thus limiting the oxygen-carrying capacity of the blood, can directly damage both myocardial cells and the arterial intima. It is more reasonable to implicate carbon monoxide in myocardial disease because of the great need of the cardiac musculature for oxygen. Since the heart is known to consume most of the oxygen available to it, any disorder that decreases the oxygen in the circulating blood could directly impair cardiac muscle metabolism. If any degree of ischemia already existed, the decrease in oxygen-carrying capacity produced by a significant increase in carboxyhemoglobin could conceivably be responsible for irreversible ischemic necrosis.

Nicotine, by increasing myocardial irritability, could trigger a fatal arrhythmia. By provoking arteriolar spasm it could also impair blood flow in the microcirculation of the heart and other organs. An effect of nicotine on platelet coagulability has been suggested, and through this mechanism cigarette smoking may play a role in thrombus formation. If so, it may be that increased rates of atherosclerosis in smokers result from incorporation of clots from the intimal surface into the intima (the pathogenesis of atheroma formation or enlargement).

The data from Framingham are certainly consistent with the concept that nicotine and carbon monoxide can be hazardous to a heart that already has been placed in jeopardy by reason of major atherosclerotic narrowing. In the individual without significant coronary narrowing, the effect of smoking may be much less deleterious. If, however, damage to the intima from any cause may be the inciting factor in the production of atherosclerosis, both nicotine and carbon monoxide may be implicated.

The decreased effect of smoking with age was also not readily explicable. Obviously the difference in the impact of smoking at various ages had an important bearing on its overall effect on coronary heart disease. The greatest effect of cigarette smoking was in the age groups in which the absolute incidence of disease was least; the effect was less as the disease incidence became higher. As a result, the difference in the incidence rates of smokers and nonsmokers was much smaller when the entire group was considered. For example, over the full time period covered the average annual incidence rate per 1,000 person-years of all coronary heart disease was 11.9 for male cigarette smokers versus 10.1 for nonsmokers. For myocardial infarction the comparative rates for men were 7.0 versus 5.8. Even for sudden death, in which cigarette smoking had the strongest relation to incidence, the average annual rate for all cigarette smokers was 2.7 versus 2.1 for nonsmokers. The apparent loss or weakening of the effect of cigarette smoking with age may be the result of a marked increase in the strength of other risk factors, including age itself. If the effect of a risk factor such as cigarette smoking were to remain constant while that of other factors were to increase with age, the *relative* effect of cigarette smoking would become less.

Another possibility is that some individuals are particularly susceptible to the effects of cigarette smoking. Only certain individuals demonstrate premature heartbeats when exposed to cigarettes. If such individuals were removed by sudden death or the development of overt disease at an early age, the remaining population at risk would be less susceptible to the effect of cigarette smoking and eventually the incidence rates in the two groups would approximate each other.

The data from Framingham are consistent with either of these hypotheses. Probably both mechanisms are at work. In any case, it is apparent that the great increase in risk of myocardial infarction and sudden death are particularly notable in younger individuals. The major benefit of quitting smoking will be found in younger persons; stopping after many years, and at an advanced age, will have little effect on atherosclerotic disease.

Diabetes and Cardiovascular Disease

12

INCLUDED IN THE HYPOTHESES to be studied in Framingham was the association of diabetes mellitus with premature atherosclerotic disease of the coronary, cerebral, and peripheral arteries. By the time plans for the Framingham Study had developed, considerable data were available that attested to a high frequency of cardiovascular disease in diabetics (Root et al., 1939; Hart, 1949). Even in the absence of carefully controlled studies there was general acceptance of the belief that, for unknown reasons, more extensive arteriosclerotic disease was found in diabetic patients than in the general population. The previous belief that hyperglycemia, especially if persistent, could damage the arterial endothelium and thus lay the groundwork for atherosclerotic change had few adherents even by 1950. Some physicians continued to accept the hypothesis that fluctuations in blood sugar might be responsible. The absence of any association between the severity of diabetes, largely measured by glucose intolerance, and the degree of atherosclerosis was important evidence against the hyperglycemia hypothesis. The relative hypercholesterolemia often observed in diabetes mellitus was considered a possible factor. Preinsulin treatment of diabetes with a high fat diet was also thought to be contributory. The hyperlipidemia and adiposity often observed in mature-onset diabetes was postulated as one of the factors responsible for the allegedly high prevalence of coronary artery disease in diabetic subjects.

Hypertension was reported to be more common than usual in persons with diabetes. The absence of solid information about the prevalence of various levels of blood pressure in the general population of nondiabetics made an estimate of hypertension in diabetics difficult. In addition, there were no firm statistics to indicate whether the increased blood pressure preceded or followed the onset of diabetes.

The relation of diabetes to cerebral vascular disease was generally discounted. However, the coronary arteries, particularly those in the lower extremity, were believed especially subject to damage by diabetes mellitus (Root et al., 1939). Studies by pathologists attested to the similarity of the pathological process in the atherosclerosis seen in diabetics and nondiabetics. Even some years after the initiation of the Framingham Study the lack of suitable control groups was recognized in attempts to compare the incidence of cardiovascular disease in the diabetic population with that in otherwise healthy persons. Expectations that the data from Framingham and similar studies would answer such questions were expressed (Liebow, Hellerstein, and Miller, 1955). In spite of the absence of good comparative data, physicians continued to believe that arteriosclerotic heart disease was more common in diabetes mellitus. However, much of this belief was based on observations in juvenile diabetes. The difference between the amount of vascular disease observed in diabetics and nondiabetics decreased with age. This observation was confounded by the rapid drop with age in the number of juvenile diabetics and a concomitant rise in the number of patients with mature-onset diabetes. The thesis that better control of carbohydrate metabolism through diet and insulin would prevent the atherosclerotic complications of diabetes mellitus gained considerable support. The late E. P. Joslin, who played a major role in the early epidemiologic studies of diabetes in Oxford, Massachusetts, was one of the strong advocates of this concept (Joslin, 1935).

More recently, interest has centered on the microcirculation. Microangiopathy has been described in numerous locations in diabetic patients, including the vaso vasorum of the major arteries (Lundbaek et al., 1970). Pathology of the small vessels has been suggested as a cause of the cardiomyopathy seen in diabetics. Congestive heart failure may be caused by a combination of large-vessel disease (the coronary arteries) and microangiopathy in the myocardium.

Criteria for the Diagnosis of Diabetes Mellitus

The need to define a prevalence and incidence case for diabetes mellitus that would be applicable to examination of an ambulatory population of apparently well people posed certain problems. The ideal approach would have involved a glucose tolerance test at each examination. At the time the study was being planned, this did not appear practicable. Collection of a fasting specimen was not considered feasible either (and furthermore might have resulted in underdiagnosis of the disease). A decision was therefore made that we would obtain random blood glucose determinations, noting the time of the last meal and its general content. Urinalyses for sugar would also be conducted. The medical history included previous information regarding any diagnosis of diabetes, hyperglycemia, or glycosuria together with any treatment regimen. Later in the study, glucose tolerance was also determined. It was decided that the category "diabetes" for this study would include all persons in whom a clinical diagnosis had been made, based on either our own clinical examination or other medical information.

Our initial examination of the population supported the experience of other studies of the prevalence of diabetes. The overall prevalence rate in the Framingham Study was 1.92 percent. Approximately half of these subjects were already aware of the diabetes diagnosis; the remainder were unaware of any abnormality. From studies earlier than ours came evidence that in some persons who had been diagnosed as diabetics it had not been possible to confirm the disease (O'Sullivan, Williams, and McDonald, 1967). However, for our purposes it seemed both reasonable and practicable to accept a clinical diagnosis of the disease from our own data or an evaluation by a private physician. On this basis we formulated an initial population at risk with diabetes mellitus to be compared with the nondiabetic population. Evaluation by medical history and random blood glucose and urine sugar examinations was repeated at each biennial examination, to determine new cases of diabetes to be included in the population at risk.

In 52 men and 47 women diabetes was diagnosed at the time of initial examination. Over the years a much larger number of subjects (397) developing diabetes was added to this population. The high number, which suggests that almost 10 percent of the population have, or will develop, this disease, may be an artifact of the all-inclusive nature of the diagnostic criteria.

Diabetes Mellitus and Coronary Heart Disease

Statistically, the development of atherosclerotic disease may be analyzed on the basis of the diabetic status at initial examination. It may also be based on diabetic status at each examination, including all individuals ever diagnosed as having diabetes mellitus. The former analysis will include only diabetics who have had the disease for an extended period of time; the latter will have many more subjects, most of whom have had the disease for only a limited time. Results of both analyses will be presented.

Based on the diagnosis determined at initial examination, coronary heart disease was observed to be definitely higher in those with diabetes than in the nondiabetics (Fig. 12-1). Similar high rates of the different manifestations of coronary heart disease, atherothrombotic brain infarction, and intermittent claudication were observed. This analysis compares the experience of subjects with diabetes mellitus with the remainder of the study population, many of whom developed this disease while under observation. Because of the high incidence of diabetes in the population after the initial examination, an analysis including all the additional cases would appear more valuable. Data presented henceforth will therefore be based on all subjects in whom a diagnosis of diabetes mellitus was ever made.

The experience of these individuals with regard to the development of coronary heart disease may be compared to that of those remaining free of diabetes (Fig. 12-2). The rate of coronary heart disease in diabetic men was clearly greater with the overall risk in the diabetics more than twice that of the nondiabetics. Among the women, diabetes posed a much greater threat. When diabetes was present in women, the risk was greatly increased and equaled that of men with this disease. When diabetic women were compared to nondiabetic women, the added risk of diabetes was very impressive—for all age groups, diabetic women had five times the risk of those without diabetes.

Diabetes Mellitus and Myocardial Infarction

The average annual incidence rates of myocardial infarction followed a similar pattern, with approximately twice the rate in diabetic men compared to those without this disorder. In diabetic women the rate was almost six times that in nondiabetic women (Fig. 12-3).

Diabetes Mellitus and Sudden Death

Owing to the small population at risk, the 24-year incidence of sudden death in the subjects diagnosed as diabetic at initial examination was too small for satisfactory analysis. However, the rates may be compared for all ages. In men, no significant difference was found. In women, although the sudden death rate was low, for women with diabetes it was three times the rate for nondiabetics (32 out of 1,000 as opposed to 11). Based on the average annual rates, which took into consideration the differences in the time during which the subjects were at risk, a stronger relation of diabetes to sudden death was observed (Fig. 12-4). The rate was approximately doubled in the diabetic men, and in diabetic women at all ages the rate was almost ten times higher. In fact, the incidence of sudden death in diabetic women was approximately that of men.

Diabetes Mellitus and Peripheral Vascular Disease

A major complication of diabetes mellitus is vascular insufficiency of the lower extremities. This is usually manifested by symptoms of intermittent claudication. Gangrene, calling for amputation of toes or even the entire leg, can be a frequent complication. Some of the problem may be attributable to small-vessel disease and atheromatous embolism from lesions on the wall of the aorta. The seriousness of the problem of peripheral arterial disease may be discerned from a review of the incidence of intermittent claudication in the Framingham population. The average annual incidence rate of intermittent claudication in men at all ages with diabetes mellitus was about five times that of the nondiabetic group (Fig. 12-5). In women the ratio was still higher (eight to nine times the rate of nondiabetic women). The greatest contrast was seen in the younger subjects (age 40-49), with a decrease in the ratio with increasing age. By age 70 in men no increase in risk was apparent; in women the added risk of diabetes still persisted.

The reasons for the particularly high risk of peripheral vascular complications in diabetes mellitus have not been established. Until recently the belief in atheromatous embolism was not widely held. Now, increasingly, neurologists are attributing cerebral vascular accidents to atheromatous emboli from the ascending aorta and neck vessels. The lower extremities are at a much greater risk. The entire length of the descending aorta and the iliac and femoral arteries are the sites of numerous atheromatous lesions. The forceful thrust of the columns of blood in these vessels, particularly the aorta, probably dislodges any incipient thrombus and some of the material in the atheromatous ulceration, driving it down the peripheral artery until it is blocked in a small arterial branch. This mechanism would account for the high susceptibility to vascular insufficiency in the lower extremity, particularly in subjects with diabetes mellitus.

Diabetes Mellitus and Atherothrombotic Brain Infarction

The risk of developing atherothrombotic brain infarction was much greater in those with diabetes than in the nondiabetic subjects. When the analysis was conducted using average annual incidence rates, the differences were marked until quite old age in both sexes (Fig. 12-6). Diabetes mellitus is an extremely potent factor in the development of atherothrombotic stroke.

Interrelationships of Risk Factors in Diabetes Mellitus

Diabetes mellitus is an important risk factor for the development of all manifestations of atherosclerotic disease. One question answerable from the Framingham data concerns the importance of any related risk factors. Comparison of a number of these in the diabetic and nondiabetic population at initial examination, or at the examination in which the diagnosis was first recorded, brings out some interesting relationships (Table 12-1). In men, except in the oldest age group, and in women in all age

Table 12-1   Risk factors in population, by diabetic status.

Diabetic status	Blood pressure		Relative weight	Cholesterol (mg %)
	Systolic (mm Hg)	Diastolic (mm Hg)		
MEN AGE 30-39				
No diabetes	131.5	83.3	100.3	216.7
Diabetes	136.0	89.4	108.6	219.2
AGE 40-49				
No diabetes	136.0	86.7	100.8	226.3
Diabetes	139.8	90.0	107.7	230.0
AGE 50-59				
No diabetes	143.2	88.2	101.5	226.1
Diabetes	144.3	87.7	107.3	231.5
WOMEN AGE 30-39				
No diabetes	123.7	78.7	96.6	203.0
Diabetes	129.5	82.8	105.7	216.6
AGE 40-49				
No diabetes	135.3	84.8	101.5	225.5
Diabetes	147.5	90.7	113.9	239.9
AGE 50-59				
No diabetes	151.7	90.3	107.2	250.8
Diabetes	161.4	94.0	119.2	253.1

groups the average blood pressure, both systolic and diastolic, was higher in those with diabetes than in those without this disorder. The differences were small but highly significant and would account for some of the effect of diabetes on atherosclerotic disease when measured in a large group.

The relative weight of the diabetic subjects, both men and women in all age ranges, was higher than in nondiabetics. The excess weight was in the range of 8-12 percent, with differences greater in the women than in the men.

Serum cholesterol levels of diabetic subjects were also higher. In men this difference was only about 5 mg %; in women it was as high as 14 mg % in the younger subjects and decreased with age. Physical activity, cigarette smoking, and uric acid levels were not significantly different in diabetics and nondiabetics.

Thus blood pressure, weight, and cholesterol levels were all higher in diabetics and played some role in determining the added risk of this disorder. A recent comparison of the high-density liproprotein cholesterol in diabetics and nondiabetics showed a lower level of this lipid fraction in the former group (Gordon et al., 1977).

(continued on page 200)

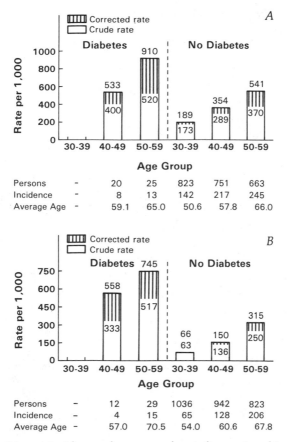

Fig. 12-1 *24-year incidence of coronary heart disease in subjects with diabetes mellitus, age 30-59 at entry. A, men; B, women.*

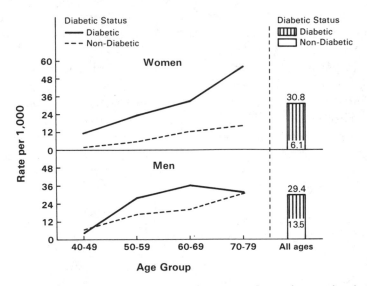

Fig. 12-2 *Average annual incidence of coronary heart disease, by diabetic status.*

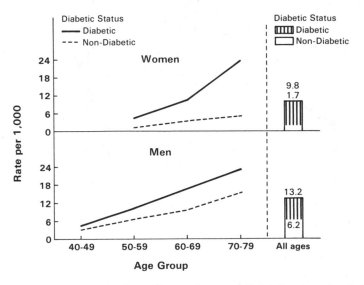

Fig. 12-3 *Average annual incidence of myocardial infarction, by diabetic status.*

DIABETES AND CARDIOVASCULAR DISEASE

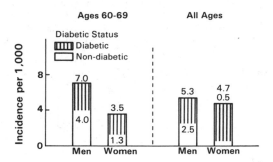

Fig. 12-4 *Average annual incidence of sudden death, by diabetic status.*

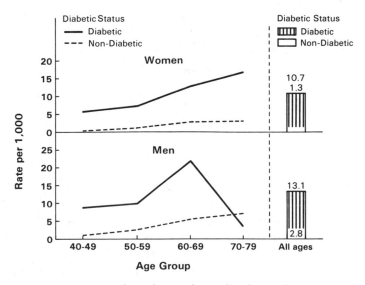

Fig. 12-5 *Average annual incidence of peripheral vascular disease, by diabetic status.*

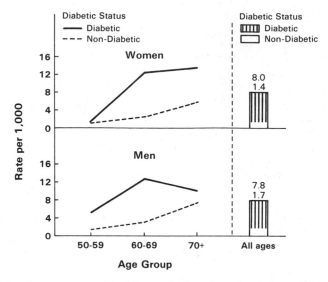

Fig. 12-6 *Average annual incidence of atherothrombotic brain infarction, by diabetic status.*

Summary

Diabetes contributes importantly to the risk of all manifestations of atherosclerotic disease, myocardial infarction, angina pectoris, sudden death, peripheral arterial disease, and atherothrombotic stroke. Although other risk factors, particularly elevated blood pressure, cholesterol level, and weight, are significantly related to diabetes, these factors do not totally explain the added risk observed in this disease.

The positive association of all manifestations of atherosclerotic disease with diabetes suggests that it is responsible primarily for acceleration of the atherosclerotic process. Concentration on the carbohydrate abnormality in diabetes, and the assumption that this was the only or the overwhelming defect, has obscured the importance of other aspects of this metabolic disease. The errors of metabolism include not only carbohydrate intolerance but faulty handling of fats and proteins as well.

The Framingham Study subjects with diabetes mellitus included all degrees of diabetic involvement. However, there were few with severe diabetes, particularly the juvenile-onset disease frequently seen in diabetes clinics. Virtually all subjects had mature-onset disease; approximately half had previously unrecognized diabetes manifested only by moderate elevation of blood sugar and possibly glycosuria. They were referred to their physicians, if not already under medical supervision. The level of medical care in the community was excellent; any complications that occurred in the diabetic Framingham subjects did so in spite of adequate control of their carbohydrate abnormalities and satisfactory general medical care.

Other Risk Factors

13

A NUMBER OF additional factors have been suggested as having an association with atherosclerotic disease, even though a positive relationship has not been established and may be controversial. In this chapter the more important of these factors will be considered.

Hemoglobin Values

Polycythemia was observed in association with thrombotic complications of atherosclerosis many years ago (Norman and Allen, 1937). Increased blood viscosity and a heightened tendency to clot formation were considered responsible. The association was with polycythemia vera and the excessively high hemoglobin and hematocrit values found in this disease. Whether the upper limits of the range of hemoglobin found in those with no diagnosable hematologic disorder were so associated also is not known.

Hemoglobin and hematocrit have been measured at each examination in the Framingham Study. Either can be used for study purposes, and as might be expected in a healthy population the range of both measurements was small. Because of the lower hemoglobin values in women, a cutoff point of 14 gm was selected, as opposed to 15 gm in men. Above these points a possible deleterious effect might be observed. When the atherosclerotic disease rates for the subjects above and below these values were compared, there was little difference. In coronary heart disease too, no significant difference was observed. When the break points were raised (for instance, to 15 gm for women), a trend appeared but the numbers of subjects involved became too small for analysis. In atherothrombotic brain infarction there was a slightly higher rate for men in the category with hemoglobin levels above 15 gm. This was associated with an age of onset three years earlier in the higher hemoglobin category. In the oldest women (Fig. 13-1) a similar difference in incidence was seen, again with an age of onset three years earlier. No significant relationship was observed in peripheral arterial disease.

From the data we may conclude that the usual range of values of hemoglobin seen in a community does not play an important role in atherosclerotic disease, with the possible exception of stroke. However, the data also suggest that excessively high values may well have some effect—although the number of persons with such aberrations, even in a large population, would be too small to have any important impact on the incidence of atherosclerotic disease.

Alcohol Intake

In the population studied, alcohol consumption was common but excessive use was not. The group with the highest consumption (100 oz or more per week) contained less than 100 men and almost no women. For this reason observations on the incidence of the atherosclerotic diseases according to alcohol consumption were limited. When such comparisons were made, no significant relationship of alcohol intake to coronary heart disease, stroke, or peripheral arterial disease was found. Within the range of alcohol consumption reported in this community, neither a deleterious nor a protective effect was observed; however, the available data do not preclude the possibility that much higher levels of alcohol consumption might have some effect.

Previous studies had indicated that the blood pressure of the men with the highest alcohol intake was several millimeters of mercury higher than that of the remainder of the population (Dawber et al., 1967). In view of the known acute effects of alcohol in raising blood pressure, the above finding is not surprising; at the time of examination, evidence of recent alcohol consumption was present in a limited number of subjects. The fact that the acute effects of alcohol consumption include a rise in blood pressure has no pertinence to the development of hypertension in the population.

Coffee Consumption

Previous reports regarding the effects of coffee consumption were confirmed by 24 years of observation (Dawber, Kannel, and Gordon, 1974; Thomas, in press). There was an association between coffee drinking and overall mortality, but coffee intake was strongly correlated with cigarette smoking. When correction was made for this correlation, no adverse effect of coffee intake was observed. Incidence rates for the various manifestations of atherosclerotic disease were in general slightly lower for those who did not drink coffee, but the differences were not statistically significant. These findings differ from those of certain retrospective studies, but are in agreement with the majority of reports (Jick et al., 1973).

From the Framingham data, within the usual range of coffee consumption no hazard for coronary heart disease, stroke, or peripheral artery disease was apparent. Too few consumers of large amounts of coffee (20 cups or more per day) were found in this population to determine any possible hazards of high levels of intake.

Cardiac Abnormalities

That evidence of cardiac abnormalities as shown by electrocardiograms or chest x-rays should be associated with an increased incidence of coronary heart disease is not surprising. Although heart enlargement by x-ray and electrocardiographic evidence of bundle branch block and left ventricular hypertrophy have been considered risk factors for the development of coronary heart disease, they may represent manifestations of previous damage to the myocardium and conduction system secondary to coronary artery disease.

For every age bracket and in both sexes the incidence of coronary heart disease was significantly higher in those subjects with x-ray evidence of myocardial enlargement (Fig. 13-2). The overall rate in men was approximately twice as high in those with heart enlargement as in those without this finding. In women the rate was almost three times higher.

The enlargement represents both dilatation of the heart chambers and hypertrophy of the muscle. The mechanisms by which ischemia could lead to the former is easily understood; the reasons for hypertrophy in the absence of elevated blood pressure are less clear. Hypertension is a frequent concomitant and precursor of heart enlargement. Even in the absence of other risk factors some individuals present with heart enlargement, which appears to carry an added risk of developing coronary heart disease.

The average annual incidence rate of atherothrombotic brain infarction for all age groups of men with heart enlargement was twice that of those without enlargement (Fig. 13-3). In women the rate was almost five times higher. Much of this could result from associated blood-pressure elevation.

Electrocardiographic Abnormalities

Left Ventricular Hypertrophy

The presence of this electrocardiographic abnormality may represent not only hypertrophy of the left ventricle but possibly damage to the myocardium because of high pressure against the ventricular wall and/or ischemia of the myocardium. It is markedly associated with elevated blood pressure. The finding of left ventricular hypertrophy by electrocardiogram is rather ominous. Average annual incidence rates of coronary heart disease were almost five times greater in those subjects, both men and women, with this abnormality (Fig. 13-4). The higher rate is observed in all age groups.

Similar ratios held true for myocardial infarction and angina pectoris. The rate of sudden death in subjects with left ventricular hypertrophy compared to those without this finding was even higher (Fig. 13-5). Clearly, left ventricular hypertrophy is an abnormality strongly associated with subsequent development of all manifestations of coronary heart disease. Not only was there a strong relationship to coronary heart disease, but also to atherothrombotic brain infarction, with an overall risk in those with this abnormality ten times that of other subjects.

Much of this effect is related to the concomitant blood-pressure elevation.

Nonspecific Electrocardiographic Changes

One of the most common electrocardiographic abnormalities involves the flattening and inversion of T waves. In the presence of S-T-segment deviation these may more clearly reflect ischemia of the myocardium. T-wave changes alone, in the absence of diagnosable myocardial disease such as a previous myocardial infarction, myocarditis, or pericarditis, have not been easy to interpret.

Analysis of this abnormality indicated that it was highly predictive of the subsequent development of coronary heart disease (Fig. 13-6). Including all subjects who had or developed nonspecific T-wave changes, average annual incidence rates at all ages and for both sexes showed two to three times the risk of coronary heart disease compared to those who never showed this change. Similar relationships were seen for other manifestations of coronary heart disease. The incidence of atherothrombotic brain infarction in the group of subjects with nonspecific T-wave change was also very high. For all ages the rates in men and women were four to five times higher than in the general population.

Left and Right Bundle Branch Block

The finding of bundle branch block on an electrocardiogram has always been difficult to interpret. The fact that this abnormality may be found following diseases in which myocarditis may occur (diphtheria, for instance) has led to an assumption that intercurrent infections may be responsible (Perry, 1939). Another possible cause is ischemia resulting from coronary artery disease. Consequently, bundle branch block may be merely an early manifestation of coronary heart disease rather than a predictor.

Analysis of the effect of bundle branch block on the occurrence of coronary heart disease requires the calculation of average annual incidence rates that take into consideration not only those presenting with this defect at the onset of the study, but also those in whom it appeared during the 24-year observation period.

OTHER RISK FACTORS

Block involving the left bundle has been considered much more important in terms of pathological significance and prognosis. Comparison of the risk of developing coronary heart disease for both men and women with and without left or right bundle branch block shows that there is a significant risk of total coronary heart disease and myocardial infarction when either left or right block is present (Table 13-1). The risk is somewhat greater in left bundle branch block in both sexes, but in right bundle branch block the added risk is certainly still important. There is no reason to conclude that the latter finding is a benign condition.

Table 13-1 Correlation of bundle branch block with coronary heart disease and myocardial infarction: average annual incidence rate over 24 years.

Left branch block				Right branch block			
Men		Women		Men		Women	
Yes	No	Yes	No	Yes	No	Yes	No
In coronary heart disease:							
32	14	34	7	25	14	19	7
In myocardial infarction:							
15	8	—	2	12	8	—	2

(continued on page 211)

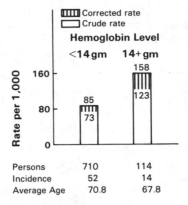

Fig. 13-1   *24-year incidence of atherothrombotic brain infarction, by hemo-globin level, in women age 50-59 at entry.*

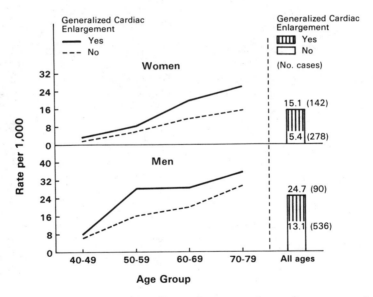

Fig. 13-2   *Average annual incidence of coronary heart disease occurring in subjects with generalized cardiac enlargement.*

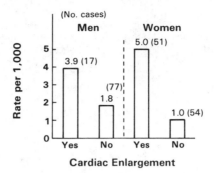

Fig. 13-3 *Average annual incidence of atherothrombotic brain infarction in subjects with cardiac enlargement.*

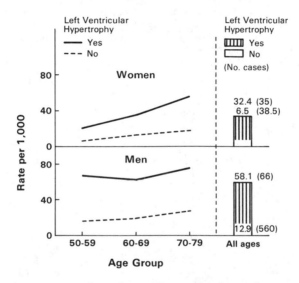

Fig. 13-4 *Average annual incidence of coronary heart disease in subjects with left ventricular hypertrophy by ECG.*

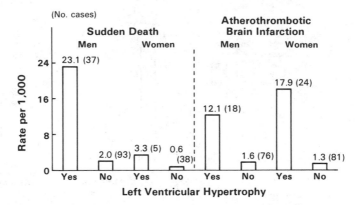

Fig. 13-5 *Average annual incidence of sudden death and atherothrombotic brain infarction in subjects with left ventricular hypertrophy by ECG.*

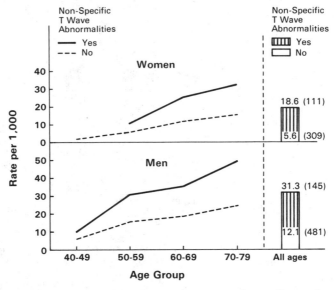

Fig. 13-6 *Average annual incidence of coronary heart disease in subjects with nonspecific T-wave abnormalities.*

Combination of Risk Factors

In many reports from the Framingham Study figures have been presented that have estimated risk on the basis of multiple factors (Kagan et al., 1963; Dawber, Kannel, and McNamara, 1964). If a given subject has high values of blood pressure, serum cholesterol, weight, cigarette smoking and/or other factors, the risk may be extremely high. In the presence of only moderate elevation but with a number of factors involved, the total risk still may be considerable.

Although estimation of risk on the basis of combinations of factors can be an interesting exercise, the use of this calculation to select those at highest risk—the top 10 percent—may also be misleading. If a cutoff point is selected above which intervention will be advised and below which nothing is advocated, a disservice may be done to a large number of people who might have benefited. Actually, the practicing physician must consider the individual risk factors and decide on the basis of each what should be done. His decision will be helped by knowledge of the degree of risk based on multiple factors, but his action should not rest solely on the estimate of total risk. Rather, the decision should be made on the basis of the need for reduction of risk and the practicability of accomplishing changes in any risk factors present. Moderate elevation of blood pressure in the presence of hypercholesterolemia may be as hazardous as much higher blood-pressure levels in persons with low serum-cholesterol levels. Eventually, however, a decision must be made whether lowering blood pressure is practicable—and, if so, by what means. Discontinuance of cigarette smoking will be of great value regardless of whether or not other risk factors are present. Excess weight should be avoided with or without hypertension. Because the approach to intervention must be made on an individual basis for each risk factor, no risk estimates are provided here for combinations of factors.

Congestive Heart Failure

14

IN ADDITION TO the immediate ischemic and thromboembolic complications of atherosclerotic disease of the coronary arteries, there is the problem of myocardial damage resulting from repeated episodes of ischemia, not sufficient individually to produce measurable lasting damage. The ultimate result of myocardial injury is congestive heart failure. This disorder was not one of the problems originally included in the Framingham design. Very clearly it was not solely—and possibly not primarily—related to atherosclerosis, although there is a close association and many of the risk factors for coronary heart disease are also related to congestive heart failure.

Most physicians are inclined to consider recurrence of the usual manifestations of coronary heart disease—myocardial infarction, angina, and sudden death—as the primary hazards once a diagnosis of coronary artery disease has been made. However, another of the prime risks experienced by the patient with coronary heart disease is failure of myocardial contractile function. With myocardial infarction there is actual loss of contractile tissue, with replacement by nonfunctioning scar tissue. The ability of the heart to act as a pump obviously is diminished every time some of the myocardium is destroyed. With recurrent infarctions the patient who survives still may have insufficient functioning myocardium and eventually will develop congestive failure.

At the time of onset of angina pectoris there may be no demonstrable myocardial disease except during the periods of ischemia. Even in the absence of a definable myocardial infarct, some irreversible damage to the heart muscle may be produced during the ischemic episode. Minute "infarctions" may occur, destroying muscle fibriles and replacing them with scar tissue. Diminished coronary blood supply may also impair contractility, even without destroying muscle. The first question we now try to answer relates to the role of coronary artery disease in bringing about congestive heart failure. As suggested above, myocardial infarction, because of loss of myocardial tissue, would be expected to contribute to congestive heart failure even assuming the remaining myocardium were completely healthy. The major concern is the effect of recurrent ischemia as seen in angina pectoris.

The average annual incidence rates of congestive heart failure in subjects with angina pectoris compared to those without angina give a definite answer to the question (Fig. 14-1). The incidence of congestive failure in subjects with symptoms of angina pectoris was markedly higher than expected, with the overall risk of congestive failure six to seven times that in the nonanginal subjects. Myocardial ischemia was obviously a potent factor contributing to the development of myocardial failure.

There has always been a strong belief that congestive heart failure not only was related to age but might well be a result of the aging process. *Presbycardia* is a term that has been used to describe this degenerative disorder (the aging heart syndrome, with failure as the prominent manifestation) (Dock, 1945). The incidence of congestive heart failure is unequivocally a function of age (Fig. 14-2). The 24-year incidence in the 50-59 age group in both sexes was approximately three times higher than that found in the youngest decade. Although not showing the same magnitude of sex difference observed in certain manifestations of coronary heart disease, congestive failure is more common in men than in women. The decreased rate in women is consistent with, although not as marked as, the lesser rate of coronary heart disease in females.

Risk Factors for Congestive Heart Failure

BLOOD PRESSURE

The recognition of the importance of blood-pressure level in the development of congestive heart failure has long been apparent in medical nosology. Hypertensive heart disease as a diagnostic category has been applied to a syndrome in which elevated blood pressure is associated initially with evidence of heart enlargement, primarily involving the left ventricle. Eventually congestive heart failure results, if some other untoward event does not supervene (cerebral hemorrhage or myocardial infarction or renal failure). The term *hypertensive heart disease* proved, however, to be a misnomer, since it implied that the only cause of the heart enlargement and eventual pump failure was the blood-pressure elevation. With hypertension there was an increase in coronary atherosclerosis, with resultant myocardial ischemia and coronary heart disease. In effect the eventual congestive heart failure was the result of both elevation of pressure per se and a damaged myocardium. The effect of elevated blood pressure on a perfectly normal myocardium can only be estimated. By the time there is evidence of failure the myocardium has been altered by age and ischemia of varying degrees, as well as by having been forced to pump blood against increased resistance. Presumably the apparent greater tolerance of elevated blood pressure in women stems from their decreased incidence of myocardial injury from the ischemia of coronary artery disease.

The magnitude of the effect of blood pressure on the development of congestive heart failure was considerable. Earlier reports from the Framingham Study have emphasized the importance of this factor (Kannel et al., 1972). After 24 years' observation, even using relatively crude clinical categories of blood-pressure level, a marked gradient of congestive heart failure incidence was apparent (Fig. 14-3). For the entire population the rate was approximately three times higher in persons classified as hypertensive than in those who were normotensive. Noteworthy are the almost identical incidence rates for both men and women in the 30-39 year cohort, but the marked differences seen in the next older decade. This may be interpreted as indicative of the comparably low rates of coronary heart disease in the younger cohort of men and women and the rapidly increasing rates of this disease observed in the older cohort of men.

When systolic blood pressure alone was used as the indicator of hypertensive level, an even more striking gradient was observed (Fig. 14-4). A similar gradient was also seen using diastolic pressure (Fig. 14-5). Blood pressure was a very strong predictor of the development of congestive heart failure at all ages and in both sexes, with the greatest difference in incidence rates seen in the younger subjects.

Blood Cholesterol Level

Other factors that contribute to the development of coronary heart disease might also be expected to affect the incidence of congestive heart failure. Evaluation of the data on the relation of cholesterol level to congestive heart failure showed there was a gradient of risk in both men and women in the 40-49 year cohort (Fig. 14-6). Although there was a suggestion of a gradient in the 30-39 year group, there were too few appropriate subjects to permit adequate analysis. No significant gradient was observed in the oldest subjects.

Cigarette Smoking

Any effect of cigarette smoking on congestive failure may result from a relation to coronary heart disease or to impaired pulmonary function or to both. Comparison of cigarette smokers and nonsmokers showed no relationship in the youngest cohort of either men or women, but a positive association in the two older cohorts for both sexes (Fig. 14-7).

Hemoglobin Level

The viscosity of the blood is one factor that determines the work the heart must perform. The greater the viscosity, the more energy must be expended to keep the blood circulating. The major factor related to viscosity is the percentage of the blood volume made up of red blood cells. An indirect measure of this is hemoglobin level. The range of hemoglobin in the healthy population is limited. Using a break point of 14 gm hemoglobin for women and 15 gm for men, we can separate the subjects into "low" and "high" categories, recognizing that the difference of the average value between the two groups is not great. The 24-year incidence rates of congestive heart failure by blood hemoglobin indicate some benefit from the lower hemoglobin level (Fig. 14-8).

Relative Weight

Just as blood-pressure level is a major factor in the prediction of congestive heart failure, weight also plays an important role (Fig. 14-9). In both men and women, as the relative-weight category increased, the incidence of congestive failure rose. In the 50-59 year age cohort the risk was three times greater in those 20 percent or more above the median weight than in those below it.

Since weight is associated with blood-pressure level, the effect of excess weight derives partially from this relationship. Because weight loss is attended by a drop in blood pressure, it should clearly be of considerable benefit in preventing premature congestive heart failure.

(continued on page 221)

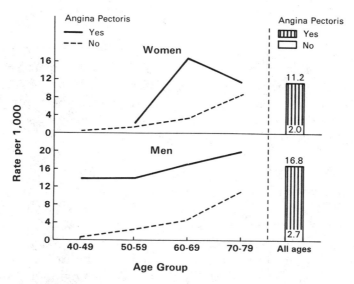

Fig. 14-1 *Average annual incidence of congestive heart failure in subjects with angina pectoris.*

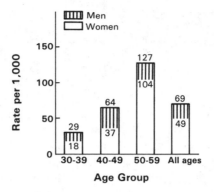

Fig. 14-2 *24-year incidence of congestive heart failure.*

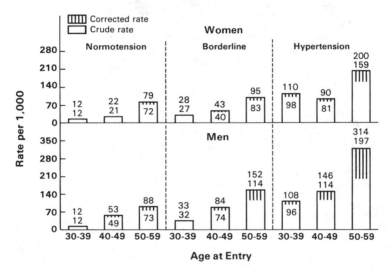

Fig. 14-3 *24-year incidence of congestive heart failure, by blood-pressure category.*

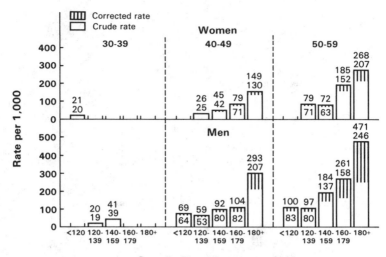

Fig. 14-4 *24-year incidence of congestive heart failure, by systolic blood pressure.*

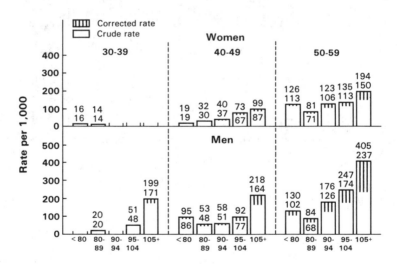

Fig. 14-5 *24-year incidence of congestive heart failure, by diastolic blood pressure.*

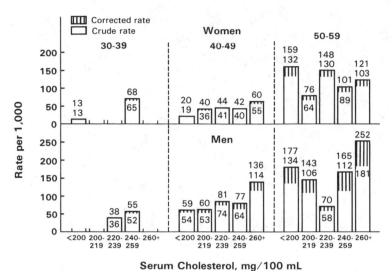

Fig. 14-6 *24-year incidence of congestive heart failure, by serum cholesterol level.*

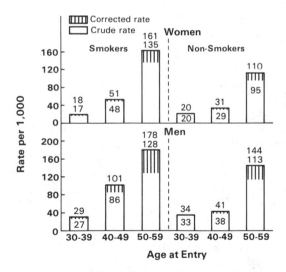

Fig. 14-7 *24-year incidence of congestive heart failure, by cigarette smoking status.*

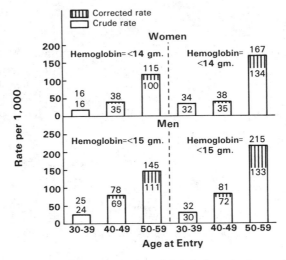

Fig. 14-8 *24-year incidence of congestive heart failure, by hemoglobin level.*

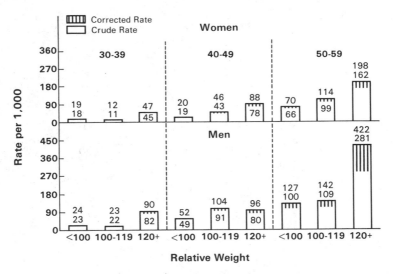

Fig. 14-9 *24-year incidence of congestive heart failure, by relative weight.*

Summary

Congestive heart failure is a common complication of all forms of heart disease. It may also be the end result of aging, in conjunction with other contributory factors of themselves not specifically considered diseases. Aging, ischemia, and the pressure against which the blood must be pumped appear to be the major factors involved.

Congestive failure is a prominent result of coronary artery atherosclerosis caused by recurrent ischemia as well as by loss of functioning myocardium resulting from infarction. A relationship to factors contributory to coronary heart disease is therefore to be expected. Blood-pressure elevation contributes to congestive heart failure not only by accelerating the atherosclerotic narrowing of the coronary artery, but also by imposing a severe burden on the heart as a pump. The strength of this factor is formidable.

High serum-cholesterol level, cigarette smoking, excess weight, and elevated blood hemoglobin are other contributing factors. If efforts to decrease the incidence of coronary heart disease were productive, they would also have a profound effect on delaying the onset of congestive heart failure—or in many instances preventing it altogether.

Impact of the Framingham Study
on Medical Practice

15

THERE OFTEN APPEARS to be a long delay between the development of new medical knowledge and its application in medical practice. Concern about this lag has been voiced particularly by those who make decisions about public appropriations for medical research. Whether the alleged delay is real and, if so, harmful is not always easy to determine; time has frequently altered our assessment of many medical therapies and surgical procedures. Reasonable delay may be distinctly beneficial to the public health.

Medical education and training are basically responsible for the attitudes of physicians toward their role in the health industry. Attitudinal change on the part of physicians, although difficult, is essential if advances are to be made in medical practice. In the past emphasis has been largely directed toward the *care of those who have already developed disease*. In spite of many contradictory claims by our medical leaders, those of us who are based in teaching institutions observe that the present generation of young physicians and trainees still sees its primary role as providing care to those who are ill. Increasingly, however, we are recognizing that prevention of disease is not merely a function of a public health department but requires action by the physician in cooperation with the individual patient.

In the past, and to a great extent even today, the efforts of medical education and training were directed toward enabling the physician to determine which of the patients coming to see him had a definable "disease" for which he had some form of treatment. Physicians went to great lengths, for example, to determine whether a myocardial infarction, no matter how small the lesion, had actually occurred. Elaborate techniques are still being devised to determine with more exactitude the size of the infarct. If a patient presents with symptoms consistent with coronary insufficiency, should the major interest center on whether some cells have or have not been destroyed? The underlying problem is advanced coronary artery disease: this is what should receive our attention.

Great interest and concern have been shown by physicians for patients with disease. If a subject turned out to be "normal," he was promptly dismissed, only to return if and when he became ill. ("Normal," in medical terminology, has been used to designate those who do not have a demonstrable disease.) A wide range of physiologic and biochemical variables in the absence of demonstrable disease was considered normal. Thus the supposedly normal range of blood pressure or blood uric acid level, for example, has been determined by measuring these characteristics in apparently healthy people—those without overt disease. As a result, the concept arose that there is "benign" hypertension, hyperuricemia, lipidemia, and many other biological variables; for a certain percentage of the so-called normal population has high values with no overt evidence of disease (stroke, clinical gout, or xanthomatosis).

Better knowledge of the natural history of the atherosclerotic process has led to a different concept of normality: that the normal person is one who not only has no disease but also is highly unlikely to develop it. At the extreme of this normality is the ideal individual who will *never* develop disease. The importance of this changing definition of normality is best illustrated by the concept of risk factors as they pertain to the development of atherosclerotic disease.

Hypertension

The association of elevated blood pressure with certain cardiovascular diseases has been recognized for many years. Congestive heart failure, aneurysm, cerebral hemorrhage, and renal failure were long noted to be more frequent in people with markedly high blood pressure. The concept of "hypertension" that most physicians have held was that of a disease associated with very high blood pressure. The most serious manifestation was that of "malignant" hypertension, in which the blood pressure rapidly increased to extreme heights associated with severe end-organ damage, often multiple. Hypertension associated with advanced renal disease, endocrine abnormalities, and congenital defects was carefully investigated to determine the basis for the underlying organic disease.

Distinguished from malignant hypertension was "benign" hypertension, which was considered to be relatively harmless unless the blood pressure began to rise rapidly. Thus watchful waiting was advocated. The level of blood pressure at which the physician should become concerned was not well defined. Diastolic pressure was considered the more important measurement —in fact, virtually the *only* one of concern.

If the distribution of blood-pressure levels of persons developing myocardial infarction and stroke over the period of the Framingham Study is examined, a wide range in both those subjects developing disease and those remaining disease free is observed (Fig. 15-1). The average value for the population continuing to remain well is to the left of that of the diseased cohort. Presumably some of those without disease will develop it. We can predict that very few of these subjects will come from the extreme left of the distribution curve. In fact, if we were to select subjects with blood-pressure levels consistently below 100/60 mm Hg, we might anticipate virtually no disease development. The blood-pressure level we should be striving to maintain is obviously much lower than what has been customarily accepted as normal. Physicians now recognize this and are taking steps to lower blood pressure in many individuals who have no stigmata of disease and who previously would not have been considered candidates for therapy.

Another enduring concept of hypertension has been that the blood pressure which best characterized an individual was the lowest that could be obtained (even under unusual and seldom attainable circumstances such as heavy sedation). Along with the expressed importance of basal pressure determination was a

IMPACT ON MEDICAL PRACTICE

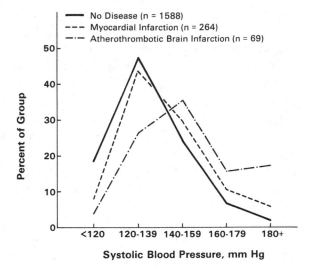

Fig. 15-1 *Distribution of systolic blood pressures of men at initial examination. The subjects later developed (1) no disease, (2) myocardial infarction, or (3) atherothrombotic brain infarction.*

belief in the inaccuracy and therefore unimportance of the casual blood-pressure determinations carried out in the usual examination in the physician's office. That the casual blood-pressure measurement is an important predictor of future disease development is one positive finding of the Framingham Study. The similarity of this measurement on repeated examinations of the same subject was quite remarkable. A single blood-pressure determination taken by a physician very accurately classified the individual compared to others of the same age and sex.

Physicians no longer dismiss an elevated blood-pressure finding as merely the result of emotional upset or other psychic factors. At the very least, such observations call for repeated measurements—which in most instances will confirm similar elevation of pressure, or at least a high degree of lability with lengthy periods of time during which the subject is exposed to an elevated pressure.

In the past the first diagnosis of hypertension frequently was made when the patient presented with congestive heart failure, angina pectoris, myocardial infarction, or stroke. The recognition that change in the size and shape of the heart as seen by chest x-ray, together with electrocardiographic evidence of left ventricular hypertrophy, is a powerful predictor of heart failure has prompted the inclusion of these studies on all hypertensive patients. Blood-pressure lowering may reverse some of these changes. In any case, the physician is alerted to the early possibility of heart failure and can institute corrective measures, such as blood-pressure lowering, weight loss, or decrease in sodium intake, prior to any clinical manifestations. The findings of a relation of elevated blood pressure to both stroke and coronary heart disease prompted clinical trials of the efficacy of antihypertensive drugs. In general, this medication has been established as beneficial, particularly in the prevention of stroke.

Lowering blood pressure relatively late in life, to the limited degree achievable, has only modest value. Instead, those developing even moderate increases of blood pressure should be sought out as early in life as possible, with the objective of preventing acceleration of this process. Certainly the medical profession is now well aware that there is no such thing as benign hypertension, and that the lower the blood pressure without actual symptoms of hypotension the better off the individual will be. Today's research increasingly emphasizes primary prevention of hypertension as the ultimate goal.

Blood Lipids

During the first half of this century, interest in blood lipids was largely confined to the investigation of persons with some obvious defect or with a known familial disease (such as familial hypercholesterolemia). People who had markedly elevated levels of blood cholesterol were highly subject to atherosclerosis and its complications. Persons not known to have a lipid disease but whose cholesterol levels were high were considered within normal limits. Data from Framingham and similar epidemiologic studies have demonstrated clearly that such elevated levels of blood cholesterol are not normal, in that they do lead to a much higher rate of coronary heart disease.

International studies have satisfactorily demonstrated that in populations in which the range of cholesterol level is considerably below that observed in Western countries, there is a much lower incidence of coronary heart disease. The Framingham Study and similar epidemiological investigations have shown that *within* the study population, the risk of coronary heart disease is also related to the individual cholesterol level compared to others in the same population. The inclusion of blood-lipid measurement in the general examination of apparently healthy people is accepted today as good medical practice. Changes in the composition of food products consistent with lowering blood-lipid levels may be responsible for some of the drop in these determinations currently being reported. Not yet clearly established are the reasons for differences in cholesterol levels within a given population. In spite of this hiatus in our knowledge, there is ample proof that dietary changes can significantly lower the serum-cholesterol level. Although the teaching of nutrition in medical school and in internships and residency programs is woefully inadequate, most physicians are reasonably well aware of what changes in diet are required.

Too often it has been the onset of clinical coronary heart disease that has brought the patient to his doctor and initiated a change in nutritional intake. The next move must be to bring the patient under medical control long before any overt disease has appeared, at a time when lipid-lowering nutrition will be most beneficial.

One development which should have taken place, but which as yet has not, is inclusion of a dietitian in the medical care of almost all patients. Dietary counsel is frequently sought in the treatment of obesity and diabetes and should be included also for persons at high risk of developing atherosclerotic disease.

Physicians more than any other group are aware of the difficulty of initiating behavioral change, and some are understandably pessimistic about efforts to accomplish it. Because of widespread resistance to dietary change, the physician has not been able to bring about the nutritional modification that is required. If present studies prove the effectiveness of cholesterol-lowering diets, changes in food preparation on a national scale would be the only practicable means of accomplishing the desired nutritional goal. Meanwhile, the current practice of large segments of the medical profession in seeking out high-risk persons and attempting through dietary means to lower their serum-cholesterol levels is a noteworthy advance in preventive medicine.

Cigarette Smoking

At the time the Framingham Study was initiated, knowledge of the relation of cigarette smoking to lung cancer was already causing many male cigarette smokers to question the wisdom of continuing this habit. When additional knowledge regarding the harmful effects of cigarette smoking on the development of coronary heart disease was publicized, the smoking habits of the population underwent noticeable change. One-third of the smokers in the middle-aged male population have given up this practice. Physicians have almost entirely abandoned cigarette smoking and strongly advocate that everyone follow their example. It is unfortunate that methods to discourage cigarette smoking completely are not more effective. The example of the medical profession is in itself one of the most potent tools. In spite of their lack of special training in behavioral science, physicians can exert great influence on their patients. The modern physician can no longer adopt the laissez-faire attitude of his predecessors toward cigarette smoking. Confronted with a relatively young male who has other characteristics suggesting increased risks of coronary heart disease, the physician is shirking his duty if he does not do his utmost to discourage the smoking habit.

Physical Activity

The Framingham Study has provided evidence of the benefit of increased-energy-output physical activity. This benefit may be related in part to weight loss, but more likely is caused by improved myocardial efficiency and metabolic change. The reaction of physicians to these findings has been similar to that relative to cigarette smoking. Many doctors participate in regular exercise and workout programs and advocate patients' making such activities part of their daily routine. A definite change in attitude toward the recovered victims of myocardial infarction has brought about early ambulation of such patients and specific encouragement for them to undertake controlled physical activity as early as possible. The medical profession is also taking an active role in advocating a change in the physical education program in schools and colleges, from organized athletics to the development of interest and proficiency in activities that can be performed throughout later life.

Obesity

A century ago the risk of death from infectious disease and other severely debilitating disorders was sufficiently high that a moderate degree of excess weight was considered medically desirable. Nutritionists advocated intake of high-calorie food by the young. The effect of this apparently "good" nutrition was to create a population in the Western countries that was overnourished and better able to withstand the infectious killer diseases of that era. The concept of desirable overnutrition has not been easy to overcome, even though the major risks of death are now those of atherosclerosis and cancer. Unfortunately, the development and progression of atherosclerotic disease is aided and abetted by the same rich diet that was so helpful in combating disease hazards a hundred years ago.

Life insurance data have long suggested that excess weight limits life expectancy. Epidemiologic studies have shown that overnutrition is a definite risk factor for certain manifestations of atherosclerotic disease. Today's physician constantly cautions against weight gain and endeavors to keep his patients well below the supposedly ideal weight of a generation or more ago.

Diabetes Mellitus

In spite of the claims of some diabetologists that the careful control of carbohydrate metabolism in diabetes will prevent atherosclerotic complications, epidemiologic studies have shown a continued high rate of these complications in the disease. Insulin and oral agents to lower blood sugar do not appear to be the full answer; not only dietary control of the carbohydrate abnormality but also attention to the quantity and quality of the fat intake is necessary. By regulating this constituent of the diet, we can definitely lessen the major complication of diabetes. Since the diabetic subject is a high-risk candidate for coronary heart disease, special attention to blood pressure, weight, physical activity, and smoking habits is essential.

In summary, it is evident that, largely as a result of epidemiologic studies in cardiovascular disease, the attitudes of the medical profession continue to change. The pessimistic view that atherosclerotic disease is an inevitable result of the aging process has been replaced by a far more optimistic concept that atherosclerosis can be prevented—or its onset significantly delayed. This can be achieved only by concern for the health of the well population long before any evidence of overt disease is apparent.

References

Publications from the
Framingham Study

Index

References

ABELL, L., B. LEVY, B. BRODIE, and F. KENDALL. 1952. A simplified method for the estimation of total cholesterol in serum and the demonstration of its specificity. *Journal of Biological Chemistry* 195:357-366.

ADLERSBERG, D., A. D. PARETS, and E. P. BOAS. 1949. Studies of families with xanthoma and unselected patients with coronary artery disease under the age of fifty years. *Journal of the American Medical Association* 141:246-254.

ALLAN, W. 1934. The relation of arterial hypertension to angina pectoris and coronary occlusion. *Southern Medical and Surgical Journal* 96:377-379.

BUNCHER, C. R. 1973. "Administratively significant." *New England Journal of Medicine* 289:155-156.

CASTELLI, W. P. 1977. Personal communication.

——, J. T. DOYLE, T. GORDON, C. G. HAMES, M. C. HJORTLAND, S. B. HULLEY, A. KAGAN, and W. J. ZUKEL. 1977. HDL cholesterol levels in coronary heart disease. A cooperative lipoprotein phenotyping study. *Circulation* 55:767-772.

COHEN, C. 1977. When may research be stopped? *New England Journal of Medicine* 296:1203-1210.

DAWBER, T. R. 1960. Summary of recent literature regarding cigarette smoking and coronary heart disease. *Circulation* 22:164-166.

——. 1973. Risk factors in young adults. *Journal of the American College Health Association* 22:84-95.

——. 1976. The interrelationship of tobacco smoke components to hyperlipidemia and other risk factors. In E. L. Wynder, D. Hoffman, and G. B. Gori, eds., *Modifying the risk for the smoker.* Washington, D.C.: Government Printing Office.

——, W. B. KANNEL, and T. GORDON. 1974. Coffee and cardiovascular disease: observations from the Framingham Study. *New England Journal of Medicine* 291:871-874.

——, W. B. KANNEL, and L. P. LYELL. 1963. An approach to longitudinal studies in a community: the Framingham Study. *Annals of the New York Academy of Science* 107:539-656.

——, W. B. KANNEL, and P. M. MCNAMARA. 1964. The prediction of coronary heart disease. *Transactions of the Association of Life Insurance Medical Directors of America* 47:70-105.

——, G. F. MEADORS, and F. E. MOORE, JR. 1951. Epidemiological approaches to heart disease: the Framingham Study. *American Journal of Public Health* 41:279-286.

——, F. E. MOORE, JR., and G. MANN. 1957. Coronary heart disease in the Framingham Study. *American Journal of Public Health* 47:4-24.

—— and J. STOKES. 1959. The silent coronary: the frequency and clinical characteristics of unrecognized myocardial infarction in the Framingham Study. *Annals of Internal Medicine* 50:1359-1369.

REFERENCES

———, H. E. Thomas, Jr., and P. M. McNamara. 1973. Characteristics of the dicrotic notch of the arterial pulse wave in coronary heart disease. *Angiology* 24:244-255.

———, W. B. Kannel, A. Kagan, R. K. Donabedian, P. M. McNamara, and G. Pearson. 1967. Environmental factors in hypertension. In J. Stamler, R. Stamler, and T. N. Pullman, eds., *Epidemiology of hypertension*. New York: Grune & Stratton.

Dock, W. 1945. Presbycardia, or aging of myocardium. *New York State Journal of Medicine* 45:983-986.

Doll, R., and A. B. Hill. 1950. Smoking and carcinoma of the lung. *British Medical Journal* 2:739-748.

Doyle, J. T., T. R. Dawber, W. B. Kannel, A. S. Heslin, and H. Kahn. 1962. Cigarette smoking and coronary heart disease. Combined experience of the Albany and Framingham studies. *New England Journal of Medicine* 266:796-801.

———, T. R. Dawber, W. B. Kannel, S. Kinch, and H. A. Kahn. 1964. The relationship of cigarette smoking to coronary heart disease: second report of the combined experience of the Albany, New York, and Framingham, Massachusetts, studies. *Journal of the American Medical Association* 190: 886-890.

Duguid, J. B. 1949. Pathogenesis of arteriosclerosis. *Lancet* 2:925-927.

English, J. P., F. A. Willius, and J. Berkson. 1940. Tobacco and coronary disease. *Journal of the American Medical Association* 115:1327-1329.

Friedman, G. D., W. B. Kannel, and T. R. Dawber. 1966. The epidemiology of gall bladder disease: observations in the Framingham Study. *Journal of Chronic Diseases* 19:273-292.

Gofman, J. W., F. Lindgren, H. Elliott, W. Mantz, J. Hewitt, B. Strisower, and V. Herring. 1950. The role of lipids and lipoproteins in atherosclerosis. *Science* 3:166-171.

Gordon, T., W. B. Kannel, D. McGee, and T. R. Dawber. 1974. Death and coronary attacks in men after giving up cigarette smoking. A report from the Framingham Study. *Lancet* 2:1345-1349.

———, W. B. Kannel, T. R. Dawber, and D. McGee. 1975. Changes associated with quitting cigarette smoking: the Framingham Study. *American Heart Journal* 90:322-328.

———, W. P. Castelli, M. C. Hjortland, W. B. Kannel, and T. R. Dawber. 1977. High density lipoprotein as a protective factor against coronary heart disease. *American Journal of Medicine* 62:707-714.

Gould, S. E. 1960. *Pathology of the heart*. Springfield, Illinois: Charles C Thomas.

Grollman, A. 1930. The action of alcohol, caffein, and tobacco on the cardiac output (and its related functions) of normal man. *Journal of Pharmacology and Experimental Therapeutics* 39:313-327.

Hart, J. M. 1949. Diabetes and arteriosclerosis. *Medical Clinics of North America* 33:795-804.

Heberden, W. 1802. *Commentaries on the history and cure of diseases*. London.

REFERENCES

HIGGINS, I. T. T., W. B. KANNEL, and T. R. DAWBER. 1965. The electrocardiogram in epidemiologic studies. *British Journal of Preventive and Social Medicine* 19:53-68.

JICK, H., O. S. MIETTINEN, R. K. NEFF, S. SHAPIRO, O. P. HEINON, and D. SLONE. 1973. Coffee and myocardial infarction. *New England Journal of Medicine* 289:63-67.

JOSLIN, E. P. 1935. *The treatment of diabetes mellitus.* Philadelphia: Lea & Febiger.

KAGAN, A., W. B. KANNEL, T. R. DAWBER, and N. REVOTSKIE. 1963. The coronary profile. *Annals of the New York Academy of Science* 97:883-894.

KAHN, H. A., H. M. LEIBOWITZ, J. P. GANLEY, M. M. KINI, T. COLTON, R. S. NICKERSON, and T. R. DAWBER. 1977. The Framingham Eye Study. I. Outline and major prevalence findings. II. Association of ophthalmic pathology with single variables previously measured in the Framingham heart study. *American Journal of Epidemiology* 106:17-32.

KANNEL, W. B., T. GORDON, and M. J. SCHWARTZ. 1971. Systolic versus diastolic blood pressure and risk of coronary heart disease—the Framingham study. *American Journal of Cardiology* 27:335-346.

―――, T. R. DAWBER, W. E. GLENNON, and M. C. THORNE. 1962. Preliminary report: the determinants and clinical significance of serum cholesterol. *Massachusetts Journal of Medical Technology* 4:11-29.

―――, E. J. LEBAUER, T. R. DAWBER, and P. McNAMARA. 1967. Relation of body weight to development of coronary heart disease: the Framingham study. *Circulation* 35:734-744.

―――, P. McNAMARA, M. FEINLEIB, and T. R. DAWBER. 1970. The unrecognized myocardial infarction—14 year follow-up experience in the Framingham study. *Geriatrics* 25:75-87.

―――, W. P. CASTELLI, P. McNAMARA, M. FEINLEIB, and P. A. McKEE. 1972. Role of blood pressure in the development of congestive heart failure. The Framingham study. *New England Journal of Medicine* 287:781-787.

KATTWINKEL, E. E., V. A. GETTING, E. M. MORRIS, and W. J. ZUKEL. 1951. Community heart program; report of 3 years' experience. *New England Journal of Medicine* 245:595-598.

KEYS, A. 1948. Nutrition in relation to etiology and course of degenerative diseases. *Journal of the American Dietetic Association* 24:281-285.

―――. 1952. Human atherosclerosis and the diet. *Circulation* 5:115-118.

―――. 1980. Seven countries: death and coronary heart disease. Cambridge, Mass.: Harvard University Press.

LEVINE, S. A., and C. L. BROWN. 1929. Coronary thrombosis: its various clinical features. *Medicine* 8:245-418.

LEVY, R. L., P. D. WHITE, W. D. STROUD, and C. C. HILLMAN. 1946. Overweight: its prognostic significance in relation to hypertension and cardiovascular renal diseases. *Journal of the American Medical Association* 131:951-953.

LIEBOW, I. M., H. K. HELLERSTEIN, and M. MILLER. 1955. Arteriosclerotic heart disease in diabetes mellitus. *American Journal of Medicine* 18:438-447.

REFERENCES

LIND, J. 1953. *Treatise on scurvy:* a bicentenary volume containing a reprint of the first edition of A Treatise of the Scurvy by James Lind, ed. C. P. Stewart and D. Guthrie. Edinburgh: University Press.

LUNDBAEK, K., V. A. JENSEN, T. S. OLSEN, H. ORSKOV, N. J. CHRISTENSEN, K. JOHANSEN, A. P. HANSEN, and R. OSTERBY. 1970. Diabetes, diabetic angiopathy and growth hormone. *Lancet* 2:131-133.

McKEE, P. A., W. P. CASTELLI, P. M. McNAMARA, and W. B. KANNEL. 1971. The natural history of congestive heart failure; the Framingham Study. *New England Journal of Medicine* 285:1141-1146.

MACKENZIE, SIR JAMES. 1926. *The basis of vital activity;* being a review of five years' work at the St. Andrews Institute for Clinical Research. London: Faber and Gwyer.

McKINNEY, B. 1974. *Pathology of cardiomyopathies.* London: Butterworths.

MANN, G. V. 1974. The influence of obesity on health. *New England Journal of Medicine* 291:178-185.

————. 1977. Diet—heart: end of an era. *New England Journal of Medicine* 297:644-650.

————, G. PEARSON, T. GORDON, T. R. DAWBER, L. LYELL, and D. SHURTLEFF. 1962. Diet and cardiovascular disease in the Framingham Study. I. Measurement of dietary intake. *American Journal of Clinical Nutrition* 11:200-225.

MARCHAND, F. 1904. Proceedings of the 21st Congress of Internal Medicine.

MARGOLIS, J. R., W. B. KANNEL, M. FEINLEIB, T. R. DAWBER, and P. M. McNAMARA. 1973. Clinical features of unrecognized myocardial infarction—silent and symptomatic. *American Journal of Cardiology* 32:1-7.

MARKS, H. H. 1960. Influence of obesity on morbidity and mortality. *Bulletin of the New York Academy of Medicine* 36:296-312.

MASTER, A. M., S. DACK, and H. L. JAFFE. 1939. Age, sex and hypertension in myocardial infarction due to coronary occlusion. *Archives of Internal Medicine* 64:767-768.

————, H. H. MARKS, and S. DACK. 1943. Hypertension in people over forty. *Journal of the American Medical Association* 121:1251-1256.

MORIYAMA, I. M. 1964. Uses of vital records of epidemiological research. *Journal of Chronic Diseases* 17:889-897.

————, T. R. DAWBER, and W. B. KANNEL. 1966. Evaluation of diagnostic information supporting medical certification of deaths from cardiovascular disease. National Cancer Institute Monograph no. 19.

NATIONAL ADVISORY HEART COUNCIL, TECHNICAL GROUP AND COMMITTEE ON LIPOPROTEINS AND ATHEROSCLEROSIS. 1956. Evaluation of serum lipoprotein and cholesterol measurements as predictors of clinical complications of atherosclerosis. *Circulation* 14:691-741.

NORMAN, I. L., and E. V. ALLEN. 1937. The vascular complications of polycythemia. *American Heart Journal* 13:257-274.

O'SULLIVAN, J. B., R. S. WILLIAMS, and G. McDONALD. 1967. The prevalence of diabetes mellitus and related variables: population study in Sudbury, Massachusetts. *Journal of Chronic Diseases* 20:535-543.

PAFFENBARGER, R. S., J. NOTKIN, E. D. KRUEGER, P. A. WOLF, M. C. THORNE,

REFERENCES

E. J. LeBauer, and J. L. Williams. 1966. Chronic disease in former college students. II. Methods of study and observations on mortality from coronary heart disease. *American Journal of Public Health* 56:962-971.

Perera, G. R. 1948. Diagnosis and natural history of hypertensive vascular disease. *American Journal of Medicine* 4:416-422.

Perry, C. B. 1939. Persistent conduction defects following diphtheria. *British Heart Journal* 1:117-122.

Petersen, O. L. 1970. The Gorgonzola diet and the prevention of myocardial infarction. In *Atherosclerosis, proceedings of the second international symposium*. New York: Springer Verlag.

Proceedings of the Association of Life Insurance Medical Directors of America. 1942. Prognosis and insurability of hypertension with particular reference to the electrocardiogram. Vol. 28, p. 18.

Root, H. F., E. F. Bland, W. H. Gordon, and P. D. White. 1939. Coronary atherosclerosis in diabetes mellitus: a post-mortem study. *Journal of the American Medical Association* 113:27-30.

Rose, G. A. 1965. Ischemic heart disease. Chest pain questionnaire. *Milbank Memorial Fund Quarterly* 43:32-39.

——, W. W. Holland, and E. A. Crowley. 1964. A sphygmomanometer for epidemiologists. *Lancet* 1:296-300.

Roth, G. M., and R. M. Shick. 1958. Effect of smoking on the cardiovascular system of man. *Circulation* 17:443-459.

Schmidt, W., and J. DeLint. 1972. Causes of death in alcoholics. *Quarterly Journal of the Study of Alcoholism* 33:171-185.

Sherman, J. F. 1977. The organization and structure of the National Institutes of Health. *New England Journal of Medicine* 297:18-26.

Smirk, F. H. 1957. *High arterial pressure*. Oxford: Blackwell Scientific Publications.

Snow, J. 1936. *Snow on cholera*. Being a reprint of two papers. (New York Commonwealth Fund). London: Oxford.

Society of Actuaries. 1959. *Build and blood pressure study*. Chicago: Society of Actuaries.

Stamler, J. 1962. Breakthrough against hypertensive and atherosclerotic diseases? Some possible implications and problems for cardiovascular research and clinical practice. *Geriatrics* 17:31-40.

Stokes, J., and T. R. Dawber. 1956. Rheumatic heart disease in the Framingham Study. *New England Journal of Medicine* 255:1228-1233.

Terris, M., ed. 1964. *Goldberger on pellagra*. Baton Rouge, Louisiana: Louisiana State University Press.

Thomas, H. E., Jr. The relationship of coffee drinking to death and cardiovascular disease. In press.

U.S. Department of Health, Education and Welfare. 1972. Vital statistics of the United States. Life tables, vol. 2, section 5. Washington, D.C.: Government Printing Office.

Vander, J. B., E. A. Gaston, and T. R. Dawber. 1968. The significance of nontoxic thyroid nodules: final report of a 15-year study of the incidence of thyroid malignancy. *Annals of Internal Medicine* 69:537-540.

REFERENCES

VIRCHOW, R. 1856. Phlogose und Thrombose im Gefassystem. In *Gesammelte Abhandlungen zur wissenschaftlichen Medicin*. Frankfurt-am-Main: Meidinger Sohn.

WHITE, N. K., J. E. EDWARDS, and T. J. DAY. 1950. The relationship of the degree of coronary atherosclerosis with age, in men. *Circulation* 1:645-654.

WILKERSON, H. L. C., and M. J. FORD. 1949. Chronic disease: diabetes control in local health department. *American Journal of Public Health* 39:607-613.

WINTER, M. D., G. P. SAYRE, C. H. MILLIKEN, and N. M. BARKER. 1958. Relationship of degree of atherosclerosis of internal carotid system in the brain of women to age and coronary atherosclerosis. *Circulation* 18:7-18.

WORLD HEALTH ORGANIZATION TECHNICAL REPORT, SERIES 168. 1959. Hypertension and coronary heart disease: classification and criteria for epidemiological studies. Geneva: WHO.

Publications from the Framingham Study

The following is a list of publications that have emanated from the Framingham Study, given in chronological order by date of publication.

1951. DAWBER, T. R., G. F. MEADORS, AND F. E. MOORE, JR. Epidemiological approaches to heart disease: the Framingham Study. *American Journal of Public Health* 41:279-286.

1952. DAWBER, T. R., AND F. E. MOORE, JR. Longitudinal study of heart disease in Framingham, Massachusetts: an interim report. *Milbank Memorial Fund Quarterly* 30:241-247 (suppl.).

1952. DAWBER, T. R., W. B. KANNEL, D. E. LOVE, AND R. D. STREEPER. The electrocardiogram in heart disease detection: a comparison of the multiple and single lead procedures. *Circulation* 5:559-566.

1954. VANDER, J. B., E. A. GASTON, AND T. R. DAWBER. Significance of solitary nontoxic thyroid nodules: preliminary report. *New England Journal of Medicine* 251:970-973.

1956. STOKES, J., AND T. R. DAWBER. Rheumatic heart disease in the Framingham Study. *New England Journal of Medicine* 255:1228-1233.

1957. DAWBER, T. R., F. E. MOORE, JR., AND G. V. MANN. Coronary heart disease in the Framingham Study. *American Journal of Public Health* 47:4-24.

1958. DAWBER, T. R., AND W. B. KANNEL. An epidemiologic study of heart disease: the Framingham Study. *Nutrition Review* 16:1-4.

1958. KANNELL, W. B., T. R. DAWBER, AND M. E. COHEN. The electrocardiogram in neurocirculatory asthenia (anxiety, neurosis or neurasthenia): a study of 203 neurocirculatory asthenia patients and 757 healthy controls in the Framingham study. *Annals of Internal Medicine* 49:1351-1360.

1959. STOKES, J., AND T. R. DAWBER. The silent coronary: the frequent and clinical characteristics of the unrecognized myocardial infarction in in the Framingham study. *Annals of Internal Medicine* 50:1359-1369.

1959. KAGAN, A., T. GORDON, W. B. KANNEL, AND T. R. DAWBER. Blood pressure and its relation to coronary heart disease in the Framingham study. *Proceedings of the Council for High Blood Pressure Research, American Heart Association* 7:53-81.

1959. GORDON, T., F. E. MOORE, D. SHURTLEFF, AND T. R. DAWBER. Some methodologic problems in the long-term study of cardiovascular disease: observations on the Framingham study. *Journal of Chronic Diseases* 10:186-206.

1959. DAWBER, T. R., W. B. KANNEL, N. REVOTSKIE, J. STOKES, A. KAGAN, AND T. GORDON. Some factors associated with the development of coronary heart disease: six years' follow-up experience in the Framingham study. *American Journal of Public Health* 49:1349-1356.

1960. DAWBER, T. R. Summary of recent literature regarding cigarette smoking and coronary heart disease. *Circulation* 22:164-166.

1961. DAWBER, T. R., W. B. KANNEL, G. PEARSON, AND D. SHURTLEFF. Assessment of the diet in the Framingham study: methodology and preliminary observations. *Health News* 38:4-6.

1961. DAWBER, T. R., AND W. B. KANNEL. Susceptibility to coronary heart disease. *Modern Concepts of Cardiovascular Disease* 30:671-675.

1961. KANNEL, W. B., T. R. DAWBER, A. KAGAN, N. REVOTSKIE, AND J. STOKES. Factors of risk in the development of coronary heart disease— six year follow-up experience: the Framingham Study. *Annals of Internal Medicine* 55:33-50.

1961. DOYLE, J. T., T. R. DAWBER, W. B. KANNEL, A. S. HESLIN, AND H. A. KAHN. Cigarette smoking and coronary heart disease: combined experience of the Framingham and Albany studies. *New England Journal of Medicine* 266:796-801.

1962. DAWBER, T. R., W. B. KANNEL, N. REVOTSKIE, AND A. KAGAN. The epidemiology of coronary heart disease—the Framingham enquiry. *Proceedings of the Royal Society of Medicine* 55:265-271.

1962. KAGAN, A., T. R. DAWBER, W. B. KANNEL, AND N. REVOTSKIE. The Framingham study: a prospective study of coronary heart disease. *Federation Proceedings* 21:52-57.

1962. DAWBER, T. R., G. PEARSON, P. ANDERSON, G. V. MANN, W. B. KANNEL, D. SHURTLEFF, AND P. McNAMARA. Dietary assessment in the epidemiologic study of coronary heart disease: the Framingham study. *American Journal of Clinical Nutrition* 11:226-234.

1962. MANN, G. V., G. PEARSON, T. GORDON, T. R. DAWBER, L. LYELL, AND D. SHURTLEFF. Diet and cardiovascular disease in the Framingham study. *American Journal of Clinical Nutrition* 11:200-225.

1962. DAWBER, T. R. Coronary heart disease: morbidity in the Framingham study, and analysis of factors of risk. *Bibliotheca Cardiologica* 13:9-24.

1962. DAWBER, T. R., AND W. B. KANNEL. Computers in epidemiologic research: uses in the Framingham study. *Circulation Research* 11:587-589.

1962. DAWBER, T. R., AND W. B. KANNEL. Atherosclerosis and you: pathogenetic implications from epidemiologic observations. *Journal of the American Geriatrics Society* 10:805-821.

1962. CORNFIELD, J. Joint dependence of risk of coronary heart disease in serum cholesterol and systolic blood pressure: a discriminant function analysis. *Federation Proceedings* 21:58-61.

1962. KANNEL, W. B., A. KAGAN, T. R. DAWBER, AND N. REVOTSKIE. Epidemiology of coronary heart disease: implications for the practicing physician. *Geriatrics* 17:675-690.

PUBLICATIONS FROM THE FRAMINGHAM STUDY

1962. KANNEL, W. B., T. R. DAWBER, W. E. GLENNON, AND M. C. THORNE. Preliminary report: the determinants and clinical significance of serum cholesterol. *Massachusetts Journal of Medical Technology* 4:11-29.

1963. DAWBER, T. R., W. B. KANNEL, AND G. D. FRIEDMAN. The use of computers in cardiovascular epidemiology. *Progress in Cardiovascular Diseases* 5:406-417.

1963. DAWBER, T. R., AND W. B. KANNEL. Coronary heart disease as an epidemiology entity. *American Journal of Public Health* 53:433-437.

1963. KAGAN, A., W. B. KANNEL, T. R. DAWBER, AND N. REVOTSKIE. The coronary profile. *Annals of the New York Academy of Sciences* 97: 883-894.

1963. KANNEL, W. B., P. BARRY, AND T. R. DAWBER. Immediate mortality in coronary heart disease: the Framingham study. *Proceedings of the 4th World Congress of Cardiology.*

1963. DAWBER, T. R., W. B. KANNEL, AND L. LYELL. An approach to longitudinal studies in a community: the Framingham study. *Annals of the New York Academy of Sciences* 107:539-556.

1964. DAWBER, T. R., W. B. KANNEL, AND P. McNAMARA. The prediction of coronary heart disease. *Transactions of the Association of Life Insurance Medical Directors of America* 47:70-105.

1964. KANNEL, W. B. Cigarette smoking and coronary heart disease. *Annals of Internal Medicine* 60:1103-1106.

1964. KANNEL, W. B., T. R. DAWBER, G. D. FRIEDMAN, W. E. GLENNON, AND P. McNAMARA. Risk factors in coronary heart disease: an evaluation of several serum lipids as predictors of coronary heart disease. *Annals of Internal Medicine* 61: 888-899.

1964. DOYLE, J. T., T. R. DAWBER, W. B. KANNEL, S. H. KINCH, AND H. A. KAHN. The relationship of cigarette smoking to coronary heart disease. *Journal of the American Medical Association* 190:886-890.

1965. KANNEL, W. B., L. K. WIDMER, AND T. R. DAWBER. Gefahrdung durch coronare Herzkrankheit; Folgerungen für die Praxis aus 10 Jahren Framingham-studie. *Schweizerische Medizinische Wochenschrift* 95: 18-24.

1965. HIGGINS, I. T. T., W. B. KANNEL, AND T. R. DAWBER. The electrocardiogram in epidemiological studies. *British Journal of Preventive and Social Medicine* 19:53-68.

1965. KANNEL, W. B., T. R. DAWBER, H. E. THOMAS, JR., AND P. McNAMARA. Comparison of serum lipids in the prediction of coronary heart disease. *Rhode Island Medical Journal* 48:243-250.

1965. KANNEL, W. B., T. R. DAWBER, AND P. McNAMARA. Vascular disease of the brain—epidemiologic aspects: the Framingham study. *American Journal of Public Health* 55:1355-1366.

1966. KANNEL, W. B., T. R. DAWBER, AND P. McNAMARA. Detection of the coronary prone adult: the Framingham study. *Journal of the Iowa Medical Society* 56:26-34.

PUBLICATIONS FROM THE FRAMINGHAM STUDY

1966. Friedman, G. D., W. B. Kannel, T. R. Dawber, and P. McNamara. Comparison of prevalence, case history, and incidence data in assessing the potency of risk factors in coronary heart disease. *American Journal of Epidemiology* 83:366-378.

1966. Thomas, H. E., Jr., W. B. Kannel, T. R. Dawber, and P. McNamara. Cholesterol-phospholipid ratio in the prediction of coronary heart disease. *New England Journal of Medicine* 274:701-705.

1966. Friedman, G. D., W. B. Kannel, and T. R. Dawber. The epidemiology of gallbladder disease: observations in the Framingham study. *Journal of Chronic Diseases* 19:273-292.

1966. Kahn, H. A., and T. R. Dawber. The development of coronary heart disease in relation to sequential biennial measures of cholesterol in the Framingham study. *Journal of Chronic Diseases* 19:611-620.

1966. Dawber, T. R., and W. B. Kannel. The Framingham study: an epidemiological approach to coronary heart disease. *Circulation* 34:553-555.

1966. Dawber, T. R., W. B. Kannel, and G. D. Friedman. Vital capacity, physical activity and coronary heart disease. In W. Raab, ed., *Prevention of ischemic heart disease: principles and practice*, pp. 254-265. Springfield, Illinois: Charles C Thomas.

1966. Kannel, W. B. Habits and coronary heart disease: the Framingham study. *U.S. Department of Health, Education and Welfare; Public Health Service publication #1515*. Washington, D.C.: Government Printing Office.

1966. Kannel, W. B. An epidemiologic study of cerebrovascular disease. In C. H. Millikan, R. G. Seikert and J. P. Whisnant, eds., *Cerebral vascular diseases. Transactions of the fifth conference held under the auspices of the American Neurological Association and the American Heart Association*. New York: Grune & Stratton.

1967. Hall, A. P., P. E. Barry, T. R. Dawber, and P. McNamara. Epidemiology of gout and hyperuricemia: a long-term population study. *American Journal of Medicine* 42:27-37.

1967. Kannel, W. B. Habitual level of physical activity and risk of coronary heart disease: the Framingham study. *Canadian Medical Association Journal* 96:811-812.

1967. Kannel, W. B., E. J. LeBauer, T. R. Dawber, and P. McNamara. Relation of body weight to development of coronary heart disease: the Framingham study. *Circulation* 35:734-744.

1967. Kannel, W. B., B. L. Tory, and P. McNamara. Epidemiology of stroke. *U.S. Department of Health, Education and Welfare; Public Health Service Publication #1607*. Washington, D.C.: Government Printing Office.

1967. Friedman, G. D., W. B. Kannel, T. R. Dawber, and P. McNamara. An evaluation of follow-up methods in the Framingham heart study. *American Journal of Public Health* 57:1015-1024.

1967. KANNEL, W. B., N. BRAND, J. J. SKINNER, T. R. DAWBER, AND P. Mc-
NAMARA. The relation of adiposity to blood pressure and development
of hypertension: the Framingham study. *Annals of Internal Medicine*
67:48-59.

1967. TRUETT, J., J. CORNFIELD, AND W. B. KANNEL. A multivariate analysis
of the risk of coronary heart disease in Framingham. *Journal of
Chronic Diseases* 20:511-524.

1967. DAWBER, T. R., W. B. KANNEL, A. KAGAN, R. K. DONABEDIAN, P.
MCNAMARA, AND G. PEARSON. Environmental factors in hypertension.
In J. Stamler, R. Stamler, and T. Pullman, eds., *The epidemiology of
hypertension*. New York: Grune & Stratton.

1967. DAWBER, T. R., AND P. McNAMARA. Coronary heart disease: identification of susceptible individuals. In R. Brest and J. Moyer, eds., *Atherosclerotic vascular disease. A Hahnemann symposium.* New York:
Appleton Century Crofts.

1967. THOMAS, H. E., JR., W. B. KANNEL, AND P. McNAMARA. Obesity: a
hazard to health. *Medical Times* 95:1099-1106.

1967. KANNEL, W. B., W. P. CASTELLI, AND P. McNAMARA. The coronary
profile: 12 year follow-up in the Framingham study. *Journal of Occu-
pational Medicine* 9:611-619.

1967. HALL, A. P. Correlations among hyperurecemia, hypercholesterolemia, coronary disease and hypertension. *Arthritis and Rheumatism*
8:846-852.

1968. DAWBER, T. R., AND W. B. KANNEL. The early diagnosis of coronary
heart disease. In *Presymptomatic detection and early diagnosis.* London: Pitman Medical Publishing Company.

1968. KANNEL, W. B., W. P. CASTELLI, AND P. McNAMARA. Epidemiology of
acute myocardial infarction. *Medicine Today* 2:56-62.

1968. KANNEL, W. B., W. P. CASTELLI, AND P. McNAMARA. Cigarette smoking and risk of coronary heart disease. Epidemiologic clues to pathogenesis: the Framingham study. *National Cancer Institute* #28:9-20.

1968. DAMON, A., S. DAMON, H. C. HARPENDING, AND W. B. KANNEL. Predicting coronary heart disease from body measurements of Framingham males. *Journal of Chronic Diseases* 21:781-802.

1968. DAWBER, T. R., AND H. E. THOMAS. Prophylaxis of coronary heart disease, stroke, and peripheral atherosclerosis. *Annals of the New York
Academy of Sciences* 149:1038-1057.

1969. KANNEL, W. B., G. PEARSON, AND P. McNAMARA. Obesity as a force
of morbidity and mortality. In F. P. Heald, ed., *Adolescent nutrition
and growth*. New York: Appleton Century Crofts.

1969. KANNEL, W. B., M. J. SCHWARTZ, AND P. McNAMARA. Blood pressure
and risk of coronary heart disease: the Framingham study. *Diseases of
the Chest* 56:43-52.

1969. HAVLIK, R. J., M. FEINLEIB, R. J. GARRISON, AND W. B. KANNEL. Blood groups and coronary heart disease: field epidemiology study. *Lancet* 2:269-270.

1969. KANNEL, W. B., AND P. McNAMARA. The evidence for excess risk in coronary disease. *Minnesota Medicine* 52:1197-1201.

1969. KANNEL, W. B., W. P. CASTELLI, P. McNAMARA, AND P. SORLIE. Some factors affecting morbidity and mortality in hypertension: the Framingham study. *Milbank Memorial Fund Quarterly* 4:116-142.

1969. KANNEL, W. B., W. P. CASTELLI, AND P. McNAMARA. Serum lipid fractions and risk of coronary heart disease: the Framingham study. *Minnesota Medicine* 52:1225-1230.

1969. KANNEL, W. B., T. GORDON, AND D. OFFUTT. Left ventricular hypertrophy by electrocardiogram: prevalence, incidence and mortality in the Framingham study. *Annals of Internal Medicine* 71:89-105.

1969. DAWBER, T. R., AND H. E. THOMAS, JR. Die Epidemiologie des Schlaganfalls. *Deutsch Medizinisches Journal* 20:33-43.

1969. DAWBER, T. R. Identification of excess cardiovascular risk: a practical approach. *Minnesota Medicine* 52:1217-1221.

1969. HALL, A. P. Observations on subjects developing a positive test for rheumatoid factor in a prospective study. *Arthritis and Rheumatism* 12-301.

1970. KANNEL, W. B., P. McNAMARA, M. FEINLEIB, AND T. R. DAWBER. The unrecognized myocardial infarction: fourteen year follow-up experience in the Framingham study. *Geriatrics* 25:75-87.

1970. DAWBER, T. R., AND H. E. THOMAS, JR. Risk factors in coronary heart disease. *Cardiovascular Nursing* 6:29-33.

1970. KANNEL, W. B., J. J. SKINNER, M. J. SCHWARTZ, AND D. SHURTLEFF. Intermittent claudication: incidence in the Framingham study. *Circulation* 61:875-883.

1970. KANNEL, W. B., P. A. WOLF, J. VERTER, AND P. McNAMARA. Epidemiologic assessment of the role of blood pressure in stroke: the Framingham study. *Journal of the American Medical Association* 214:301-310.

1970. KANNEL, W. B., T. GORDON, W. P. CASTELLI, AND J. P. MARGOLIS. Electrocardiographic left ventricular hypertrophy and risk of coronary heart disease: the Framingham study. *Annals of Internal Medicine* 72:813-822.

1970. KANNEL, W. B. Physical exercise and lethal atherosclerotic disease. *New England Journal of Medicine* 282:1153.

1970. DAWBER, T. R., AND H. E. THOMAS, JR. Environmental factors in hypertension. *Merck Monograph on Hypertension #10.*

1970. GORDON, T., AND W. B. KANNEL. The Framingham, Massachusetts, study 20 years later. In H. Kessler and J. Levin, eds., *The community as an epidemiological laboratory: a casebook of community studies.* Baltimore: Johns Hopkins Press.

1971. KANNEL, W. B., T. GORDON, AND M. J. SCHWARTZ. Systolic versus diastolic blood pressure and risk of coronary disease: the Framingham study. *American Journal of Cardiology* 27:335-346.

1971. KANNEL, W. B., W. P. CASTELLI, T. GORDON, AND P. McNAMARA. Serum cholesterol, lipoproteins, and risk of coronary heart disease: the Framingham study. *Annals of Internal Medicine* 74:1-12.

1971. KANNEL, W. B., AND D. SHURTLEFF. The natural history of arteriosclerosis obliterans. *Peripheral Vascular Disease* 3:37-52.

1971. KANNEL, W. B., T. GORDON, P. SORLIE, AND P. McNAMARA. Physical activity and coronary vulnerability: the Framingham study. *Cardiology Digest* 6:28-40.

1971. KANNEL, W. B., M. J. GARCIA, P. McNAMARA, AND G. PEARSON. Serum lipid precursors of coronary heart disease. *Human Pathology* 2: 129-151.

1971. KANNEL, W. B. The origins and evils of essential hypertension. *New England Journal of Medicine* 284:444-445.

1971. GORDON, T., AND W. B. KANNEL. Premature mortality from coronary heart disease: the Framingham study. *Journal of the American Medical Association* 215:1617-1625.

1971. CASTELLI, W. P., AND R. F. MORAN. Lipid studies for assessing the risk of cardiovascular disease and hyperlipidemia. *Human Pathology* 2: 154-164.

1971. TRUETT, J., AND P. SORLIE. Changes in successive measurements and the development of disease: the Framingham study. *Journal of Chronic Diseases* 24:349-361.

1971. McKEE, P. A., W. P. CASTELLI, P. McNAMARA, AND W. B. KANNEL. The natural history of congestive heart failure: the Framingham study. *New England Journal of Medicine* 285:1141-1146.

1971. KANNEL, W. B., P. SORLIE, AND P. McNAMARA. The relation of physical activity to coronary heart disease: the Framingham study. In O. A. Larson and R. O. Malmborg, eds., *Coronary heart disease and physical fitness*. Stockholm: Scandinavian University Press.

1971. KANNEL, W. B., F. W. BLAISDELL, R. GIFFORD, W. HASS, F. McDOWELL, J. S. MEYER, C. H. MILLIKAN, L. E. RENTZ, AND R. SELTZER. Risk factors in stroke due to cerebral infarction. *Stroke* 2:423-428.

1971. KANNEL, W. B. Current status of the epidemiology of brain infarction associated with occlusive arterial disease. *Stroke* 2:295-318.

1971. KANNEL, W. B. Habits and coronary heart disease. In E. Palmore, ed., *Prediction of life span—recent findings*. Boston: D. C. Heath and Company.

1971. KANNEL, W. B. Lipid profile and the potential coronary victim. *American Journal of Clinical Nutrition* 24:1074-1081.

1971. KANNEL, W. B., W. P. CASTELLI, J. VERTER, AND P. McNAMARA. Relative importance of factors of risk in the pathogenesis of coronary heart disease: the Framingham study. In H. I. Russek and B. I. Zohman, eds., *Coronary heart disease*. Philadelphia: J. P. Lippincott Company.

1971.   KANNEL, W. B. Medical evaluation for physical exercise programs. In P. L. Morse, ed., *Exercise and the heart*. Philadelphia: Charles C Thomas Publishing Company.

1972.   GORDON, T., AND W. B. KANNEL. Multiple contributors to coronary risk: implications for screening and prevention. *Journal of Chronic Diseases* 25:561-565.

1972.   GORDON, T., AND W. B. KANNEL. Predisposition to atherosclerosis in the head, heart, and legs: the Framingham study. *Journal of the American Medical Association* 221:661-666.

1972.   DAWBER, T. R., AND W. B. KANNEL. Current status of coronary prevention: lessons from the Framingham study. *Preventive Medicine* 1:499-512.

1972.   KANNEL, W. B., AND M. FEINLEIB. Natural history of angina pectoris in the Framingham study. *American Journal of Cardiology* 29:154-163.

1972.   KANNEL, W. B., AND T. R. DAWBER. Atherosclerosis as a pediatric problem. *Journal of Pediatrics* 80:544-554.

1972.   KANNEL, W. B., AND W. P. CASTELLI. The Framingham study of coronary disease in women. *Medical Times* 100:173-175.

1972.   KANNEL, W. B., W. P. CASTELLI, P. MCNAMARA, M. FEINLEIB, AND P. A. MCKEE. The role of blood pressure in the development of congestive heart failure: the Framingham study. *New England Journal of Medicine* 287:781-787.

1972.   KANNEL, W. B., AND T. R. DAWBER. Contributors to coronary risk, implications for prevention and public health: the Framingham study. *Heart and Lung* 1:797-810.

1972.   GORDON, T., W. B. KANNEL, P. A. WOLF, AND P. MCNAMARA. Hemoglobin and the risk of cerebral infarction: the Framingham study. *Stroke* 3:409-420.

1973.   KANNEL, W. B. Obesity and coronary heart disease. Committee on Nutrition, American Heart Association 1:1-4.

1973.   WOLF, P. A., W. B. KANNEL, P. MCNAMARA, AND T. GORDON. The role of impaired cardiac function in atherothrombotic brain infarction: the Framingham study. *American Journal of Public Health* 63:52-58.

1973.   KANNEL, W. B., AND D. SHURTLEFF. Cigarettes and the development of intermittent claudication: the Framingham study. *Geriatrics* 28:61-68.

1973.   DAWBER, T. R., H. E. THOMAS, JR., AND P. MCNAMARA. Characteristics of the dicrotic notch of the arterial pulse wave in coronary heart disease. *Angiology* 24:244-255.

1973.   MARGOLIS, J. R., W. B. KANNEL, M. FEINLEIB, T. R. DAWBER, AND P. MCNAMARA. Clinical features of the unrecognized myocardial infarction—silent and symptomatic—18 year follow-up: the Framingham study. *American Journal of Cardiology* 32:1-7.

1973. KANNEL, W. B., AND T. R. DAWBER. Hypertensive cardiovascular disease: the Framingham study. In G. Onesti, K. E. Kim, and J. Moyer, eds., *Hypertension: mechanisms and management.* New York: Grune & Stratton.

1973. GORDON, T., AND W. B. KANNEL. The effects of overweight on cardiovascular diseases. *Geriatrics* 28:80-88.

1974. KANNEL, W. B. The role of cholesterol in coronary atherogenesis. *Medical Clinics of North America* 58:363-379.

1974. GARCIA, M. J., P. McNAMARA, T. GORDON, AND W. B. KANNEL. Morbidity and mortality in diabetics in the Framingham population: 16 year follow-up study. *Diabetes* 23:105-111.

1974. KANNEL, W. B., J. M. SEIDMAN, W. FERCHO, AND W. P. CASTELLI. Vital capacity and congestive heart failure: the Framingham study. *Circulation* 49:1160-1166.

1974. KANNEL, W. B. The role of lipids and blood pressure in the development of coronary heart disease: the Framingham study. *Giornale Italia Cardiologie* 4:123-137.

1974. KANNEL, W. B., M. HJORTLAND, AND W. P. CASTELLI. Role of diabetes in congestive heart failure: the Framingham study. *American Journal of Cardiology* 34:29-34.

1974. DAWBER, T. R., W. B. KANNEL, AND T. GORDON. Coffee and cardiovascular disease: observations from the Framingham study. *New England Journal of Medicine* 291:871-874.

1974. ASHLEY, F. W., JR., AND W. B. KANNEL. Relation of weight change to changes in atherogenic traits: the Framingham study. *Journal of Chronic Diseases* 27:103-114.

1974. GORDON, T., M. R. GARCIA-PALMIERI, A. KAGAN, W. B. KANNEL, AND J. SCHIFFMAN. Differences in coronary heart disease in Framingham, Honolulu and Puerto Rico. *Journal of Chronic Diseases* 27:329-344.

1974. KANNEL, W. B., T. GORDON, AND T. R. DAWBER. Role of lipids in the development of brain infarction: the Framingham study. *Stroke* 5: 679-685.

1974. GORDON, T., W. B. KANNEL, D. McGEE, AND T. R. DAWBER. Death and coronary attacks in men after giving up cigarette smoking. *Lancet* 2:1345-1349.

1974. PEABODY, C. N., W. B. KANNEL, AND P. McNAMARA. Intermittent claudication, surgical significance. *Archives of Surgery* 109:693-697.

1975. KANNEL, W. B., J. T. DOYLE, P. McNAMARA, P. QUICKENTON, AND T. GORDON. Precursors of sudden coronary death; factors related to the incidence of sudden death. *Circulation* 51:606-613.

1975. ASHLEY, F., W. B. KANNEL, P. D. SORLIE, AND R. MASSON. Pulmonary function: relation to aging, cigarette habit, and mortality: the Framingham study. *Annals of Internal Medicine* 28:739-745.

1975. KANNEL, W. B., P. A. WOLF, AND T. R. DAWBER. An evaluation of the epidemiology of atherothrombotic brain infarction. *Milbank Memo-*

rial Fund Quarterly 53:405-448.

1975. GRESHAM, G. E., T. E. FITZPATRICK, P. A. WOLF, P. MCNAMARA, W. B. KANNEL, AND T. R. DAWBER. Residual disability in survivors of stroke—the Framingham study. *New England Journal of Medicine* 293:954-956.

1975. HJORTLAND, M. C., P. MCNAMARA, AND W. B. KANNEL. Some atherogenic concomitants of menopause: the Framingham study. *American Journal of Epidemiology* 103:304-311.

1975. DAWBER, T. R. Risk factors for atherosclerotic disease: current concepts. Upjohn.

1975. SACKS, F. M., W. P. CASTELLI, A. DONNER, AND E. H. KASS. Plasma lipids and lipoproteins in vegetarians and controls. *New England Journal of Medicine* 292:1148-1151.

1975. GORDON, T., W. B. KANNEL, T. R. DAWBER, AND D. MCGEE. Changes associated with quitting cigarette smoking: the Framingham study. *American Heart Journal* 90:322-328.

1975. FEINLEIB, M., W. B. KANNEL, R. J. GARRISON, P. MCNAMARA, AND W. P. CASTELLI. The Framingham offspring study. Design and preliminary data. *Preventive Medicine* 4:518-525.

1976. KANNEL, W. B., AND T. R. DAWBER. Misconceptions about hypertension. *Primary Cardiology* 2:4-7.

1976. KANNEL, W. B., D. MCGEE, AND T. GORDON. A general cardiovascular risk profile: the Framingham study. *American Journal of Cardiology* 38:46-51.

1976. DOYLE, J. T., W. B. KANNEL, P. MCNAMARA, P. QUICKENTON, AND T. GORDON. Factors related to suddenness of death from coronary disease: combined Albany-Framingham studies. *American Journal of Cardiology* 37:1073-1078.

1976. KANNEL, W. B. Modest blood pressure rises can be dangerous. *Hypertension* 2:16-17.

1976. KANNEL, W. B. Some lessons in cardiovascular epidemiology from Framingham. *American Journal of Cardiology* 37:269-282.

1976. GORDON, T., AND W. B. KANNEL. Obesity and cardiovascular disease: the Framingham study. *Clinics in Endocrinology and Metabolism* 5:367-375.

1976. KANNEL, W. B., T. R. DAWBER, P. SORLIE, AND P. A. WOLF. Components of blood pressure and risk of atherothrombotic brain infarction: the Framingham study. *Stroke* 7:327-331.

1976. KANNEL, W. B., D. MCGEE, AND T. GORDON. A general cardiovascular risk profile: the Framingham study. *American Journal of Cardiology* 38:46-51.

1976. KANNEL, W. B. Prevention of cardiovascular disease. *Current Problems in Cardiology* 1:1-68.

1976. GARRISON, R. J., R. J. HAVLIK, R. B. HARRIS, M. FEINLEIB, W. B. KAN-

NEL, AND S. J. PADGETT. ABO blood group and cardiovascular disease —the Framingham study. *Atherosclerosis* 25:311-318.

1976. KANNEL, W. B. Coronary risk factors. I. Recent highlights from the Framingham study. *Australia-New Zealand Journal of Medicine* 6: 373-386.

1976. KANNEL, W. B. Coronary risk factors. II. Prospects for prevention of atherosclerosis in the young. *Australia-New Zealand Journal of Medicine* 6:410-419.

1976. DAWBER, T. R., P. A. WOLF, H. E. THOMAS, T. COLTON, AND R. NICKERSON. Epidemiology of cerebral accidents due to atherosclerosis. In P. Castaigne, F. L'Hermitte, and J. Gautier, eds., *Maladies vasculaires cérébrales. Conférences de la Salpêtrière*, Paris: J. B. Baillière.

1976. KANNEL, W. B., M. C. HJORTLAND, P. MCNAMARA, AND T. GORDON. Menopause and risk of cardiovascular disease: the Framingham study. *Annals of Internal Medicine* 85:447-452.

1976. DAWBER, T. R. Erfahrungen aus der Framingham Studie—25 Jahre Framingham. *Herz-Kreisl* 8:615-620.

1977. KAHN, H. A., H. M. LEIBOWITZ, J. P. GANLEY, M. M. KINI, T. COLTON, R. S. NICKERSON, AND T. R. DAWBER. The Framingham eye study. II. Association of ophthalmic pathology with single variables previously measured in the Framingham heart study. *American Journal of Epidemiology* 106:33-41.

1977. KANNEL, W. B. Preclinical ECG precursors of cardiovascular disease. *Primary Cardiology* 3:27-31.

1977. GORDON, T., W. P. CASTELLI, M. C. HJORTLAND, W. B. KANNEL, AND T. R. DAWBER. Diabetes, blood lipids, and the role of obesity in coronary heart disease risk for women: the Framingham study. *Annals of Internal Medicine* 87:393-397.

1977. DAWBER, T. R., P. A. WOLF, T. COLTON, AND R. J. NICKERSON. Risk factors: comparison of the biological data in myocardial and brain infarctions. In K. J. Zulch, W. Kaufmann, K. A. Hossman, and V. Hossmann, eds., *Brain and heart infarct*. Berlin: Springer-Verlag.

1977. SCHNEIDER, J. F., H. E. THOMAS, JR., AND W. B. KANNEL. Precordial T wave vectors in the detection of coronary heart disease. The Framingham study. *American Heart Journal* 94:568-572.

1977. GORDON, T., W. P. CASTELLI, M. C. HJORTLAND, W. B. KANNEL, AND T. R. DAWBER. Predicting coronary heart disease in middle-aged and older persons. The Framingham study. *Journal of the American Medical Association* 238:497-499.

1977. GORDON, T., W. P. CASTELLI, M. C. HJORTLAND, W. B. KANNEL, AND T. R. DAWBER. High density lipoprotein as a protective factor against coronary heart disease. The Framingham study. *American Journal of Medicine* 62:707-714.

1977. KANNEL, W. B. Office estimation of coronary vulnerability. *Medical Digest* 23:11-15.

1977. WILLIAMS, R. R., K. R. McINTIRE, T. A. WALDMANN, M. FEINLEIB, V. L. W. GO, W. B. KANNEL, T. R. DAWBER, W. P. CASTELLI, AND P. McNAMARA. Tumor-associated antigen levels (carcinoembryonic antigen, human chorionic gonadotropin, and alpha-fetoprotein) antedating the diagnosis of cancer in the Framingham study. *Journal of the National Cancer Institute* 58:1547-1551.

1977. KANNEL, W. B. Diuretics and serum cholesterol. *Lancet* 1:1362-1363.

1977. DAWBER, T. R. Le café et les maladies cardiovasculaires. *Cahiers Médicaux* 3:463-464.

1977. WOLF, P. A., T. R. DAWBER, H. E. THOMAS, T. COLTON, AND W. B. KANNEL. The epidemiology of stroke. In R. A. Thompson and J. R. Green, eds., *Advances in neurology*, vol. 16—*Stroke*. New York: Raven Press.

1977. KAHN, H. A., H. M. LEIBOWITZ, J. P. GANLEY, M. M. KINI, T. COLTON, R. S. NICKERSON, AND T. R. DAWBER. The Framingham eye study. I. Outline and major prevalence findings. *American Journal of Epidemiology* 106:17-32.

1978. KANNEL, W. B., P. A. WOLF, AND T. R. DAWBER. Hypertension and cardiac impairments increase stroke risk. *Geriatrics* 33:71-83.

1978. WOLF, P. A., T. R. DAWBER, H. E. THOMAS, JR., AND W. B. KANNEL. Epidemiologic assessment of chronic atrial fibrillation and risk of stroke: the Framingham study. *Neurology* 28:973-977.

1978. WOLF, P. A., T. R. DAWBER, AND W. B. KANNEL. Heart disease as a precursor of stroke. In B. Schoenberg, ed., *Advances in neurology*. New York: Raven Press.

1978. WOLF, P. A., W. B. KANNEL, AND T. R. DAWBER. Epidemiology of stroke: the Framingham study. In B. Schoenberg, ed., *Advances in neurology*. New York: Raven Press.

Index

Abell, L., 124
Abell-Kendall method, 124
Adiposity, 143-145, 156. *See also* Fat
  intake
Adlersberg, D., 55
Age: and coronary heart disease, 54-
  55; incidence of atherosclerosis by,
  62-75; comparison of stroke and
  coronary heart disease by, 68; and
  blood pressure, 83-84, 89, 91, 96,
  97-98, 107, 109; and serum cholesterol, 129-132; and weight, 142-
  143, 146-148; and weight, relation
  to other risk factors, 154-156; and
  physical activity, 161-162; and
  smoking, 174-178, 187-189; and
  diabetes, 191, 194-195; and other
  risk factors, 202-211; and congestive heart failure, 213-221
Alcohol use, 56-57, 203-204
Allan, W., 92
Allen, E. V., 202
American Heart Association, 139
Anemia, 33-34
Angina pectoris: as diagnostic category, 33, 35-38; electrocardiogram
  in, 36-37; questionnaire for, 37-38;

incidence by age and sex, 64, 67;
relation to other atherosclerotic
disease, 70, 73-75; relation to
blood pressure, 95, 98; and serum
cholesterol, 131; and weight, 146,
150; and physical activity, 158,
161-162, 168; and cigarette smoking, 178; and left ventricular
hypertrophy, 205; and congestive
heart failure, 213
Antihypertensive therapy, 86-89,
  119-120, 226
Arterial lumen, 94
Atheromatous lesion, 121
Atherosclerotic cerebral vascular
  disease, *see* Cerebral vascular
  disease
Atherosclerotic disease: epidemiology, 9-13; diagnostic categories,
  30-52; hypotheses, 53-58; incidence, 59-75; types and interrela-
  tionships, 70-71, 73-75; and blood
  pressure, 119-120; and lipids, 121-
  141; and obesity, 142-156; and
  physical activity, 160-170; and
  diabetes, 190, 200-201; and other
  risk factors, 202-211